After a Lifetime of Diet Failures

Finally a Glimmer of Hope

Shannon Paul

ISBN: 1478309857
ISBN-13: 978-1478309857

Cover photograph design by Sarah Sienna

Library of Congress: 2012913816
CreateSpace Independent Publishing Platform
Charleston, South Carolina. USA

DISCLAIMER

THE CONTENTS OF THIS BOOK IS NOT TO BE CONSTRUED AS MEDICAL DIAGNOSIS, TREATMENT, ADVICE OR CLAIM, NOR IS IT INTENDED AS A SUBSTITUTE FOR A PHYSICIANS CARE. CONSULT A PHYSICIAN OR OTHER HEALH CARE PROVIDER BEFORE STARTING ANY WEIGHT LOSS OR EXERCISE PROGRAM. THE AUTHORS RESULTS ARE NOT TYPICAL. DO NOT ATTEMPT TO DUPLICATE WHAT IS WRITTEN IN THIS BOOK.

DEDICATION

To my father Richard who passed away Nov 11th 2010 at the age of 89. I don't think he liked the idea of what I was attempting here, but he enjoyed listening to my stories of where I went and the people I met. You are missed by many.

Contents

Introduction

My weight over the years has gone up and down more times than a hookers pants. Obesity in North America seems to be the curse of this century, and I've suffered with this curse in the current century as well as part of the last one.

And what's the solution other than eating less and moving more? Diet plans, pills, TV programs, videos, books, hypnotism, join the gym, buy exercise equipment and on and on. Yes, join the gym, go a half dozen times if you're lucky, and never be seen there again. Buy exercise equipment and use it the same half dozen times, then under the bed or in the garage it goes.

No jokes or well-meaning prods from friends, family or total strangers will work, nor will finding yourself in situations embarrassing or otherwise until you decide enough is enough.

I came to that point regarding another significant problem in my life, alcoholism. Nothing my family, friends, and co-workers said mattered. They were always wrong and I was always right. My drinking didn't bother anyone. How could it? Sound familiar? And you can apply that thinking to any of the addictions currently available.

I had my own ideas of what the top five addictions are in North America and I was way off. For one thing, the list seems to have ballooned to ten, but I'm sticking to 5. Old school person that I am, I thought in no particular order they would be food, alcohol, drugs, gambling and sex. Google the "top 5 addictions in North America" and see what comes up. It's very surprising.

As far as my list goes, food and alcohol addictions I have down pat. Drugs always scared me and I managed to steer clear of them. Gambling never really interested me and a sex addiction was never a possibility due to a serious lack of volunteers.

I finally gave up alcohol on March 21st 2001. I'd ended up a binge drinker who could put away 40 ounces of whisky in a 24 hour period. Most sane people know that can't be good for you.

I found this quote on the internet: "Binge drinking has the propensity to result in brain damage faster as well as more severely than chronic 'nonstop' drinking(alcoholism) due to the neurotoxic effects of the repeated rebound withdrawal effects." Well duh!! That explains much. I'm always looking for a good excuse when I do stupid things.

So for many reasons, enough was finally enough and as I sit and write this, I'm over 11 years sober. And that is pretty much the only thing I've ever stuck to in my life. But now it's time to lose the excess pounds. I started my journey into the weight loss realm in July 2003 and that is where this book starts.

I've reached a point in my life where I'm tired of carrying all this extra weight around. Feeling so damn tired all the time and I won't even get into health issues, that's going to come later. On top of that, I still smoke. After 42 years that's something else that's going to have to come to an end. Oh, so much to do and so little time.

In my mind, I want to go down from my current 300+ lbs to something manageable. I know I'll never have a size 30 inch waist again and I don't want to end up looking like a body builder type. I'm way too lazy to go through all that, but I'd be happy with some improvement of any kind. And besides, with this plan I get to go to lots of different places.

Most people dream of taking "all-inclusive" vacations, mine ended up being "all-excluded."

Origins of my Master Plan

"Here I sit on May 20th 2003 resurrecting an idea I had long before a particular reality television show."

That was the first sentence I wrote in my previous book about giving my so called master plan a shot. That book was published in Jan 2004 and I've condensed it here to less than half of what it was (I took all the boring stuff out) as well as added seven new stories in my quest to make this crazy scheme work. Nobody can say I didn't try my best.

I came up with this plan in 1992 to stick myself somewhere isolated, make the source of my problems unavailable and I'd be cured. At that time, my number one problem was alcohol. Go somewhere for 30 days with no alcohol available and hopefully, no more problem. Sounds fantastic in theory, but would it work in real life? There was only one way to find out and that's do it!

My primary location of choice was Tahiti. It sounded exotic and far away. In my booze filled world, I thought I could pull this off and then reality set in. I separated from my wife and my Tahiti plan went right out the window. I was free. Never mind quitting drinking, maybe I'd take it up a degree or two or ten. The alcohol fueled years between 1992 and 2001 were interesting. I'm surprised I'm still alive.

Resurrection of my Master Plan

So now we go to 2002. In August of that year, finding myself sober for just over a year, I bought a 15 day Greyhound bus pass valid anywhere in North America. I crossed the border from Windsor, Ontario into Detroit, Michigan and from there travelled 7000 miles, through 220 cities and towns in 13 states. It was quite a grueling trip, to say the least, but well worth doing. Once!

"…breast implants and roller blades…"

After several stops, I ended up in Los Angeles California. I grabbed a cab to Hollywood and found a cheap motel five blocks from Hollywood & Vine. I took a walk around and found one of those bus tour places. The only place I was genuinely interested in seeing was Venice Beach. I'd seen it so many times on TV and I had to go there. After touring through Beverly Hills, Rodeo Drive and other tourist spots, there before me was Venice Beach. I'd found the home of breast implants and roller blades, and both were in abundance I might add.

I splashed around in the ocean for a bit and then sat on a grassy knoll watching the babes go by. As I sat there staring at them and occasionally at the ocean, I started thinking Tahiti was out there somewhere. Suddenly my idea of sticking myself in an isolated spot for an alcohol cure came back to me. Since I'd taken care of that problem, maybe I could do it as a weight loss program. My idea was reborn!

The Search for a Location

I started searching for a location on May 22nd 2003. My number one location of choice Tahiti is out! Way too expensive. I checked out the Bahamas, but they don't want you camping there. They would prefer you stay in an expensive hotel. I thought for about two seconds going into Northern Ontario, black fly and mosquito country. No way to that! So I started looking at Central America and set my sights on Costa Rica. It's not expensive and not a long flight. Done! Costa Rica it is.

After some internet searching, I decided on a place called Santa Rosa National Park. In my time frame, it's the rainy season there and usually deserted. We shall see. And finally......

"...failure is my middle name..."

My plan in the beginning of this was to try and live off the land. I assumed in a tropical setting it should not be a problem to find foods like bananas, coconuts, fish or whatever. But you know what they always say, never assume anything.

As you read about the places I went and the situations I found myself in, remember that everything was written with pencil and paper. I tried to keep the flavor of what I'd written when I transcribed it here. So if you find me wandering, repeating myself, using short forms and an abundance of exclamation points, it's what I was feeling at the time. Blame it on slow starvation, nicotine withdrawal or medical issues. All three either at once or separately played a major or minor role in how I wrote this, what I went through and the resulting calamities I found myself in.

Also, as I wrote this, it appears I switch back and forth between metric and imperial measurement. A lot! I still see things in Fahrenheit, miles and gallons, but Canada switched to the metric system back in the 1970's and never asked me my opinion. I personally believe the switch was made for the sole purpose of enabling the government to tax the hell out of gasoline and nobody would really notice and future generations would have no clue what they are paying for gas. Today, a $1.30 a liter sounds way better than $5.85 a gallon. Anyway....................

Weight loss books are written with the goal of you ending up being successful if you follow them. Not this book, failure is my middle name. Mind you, towards the end things started looking up.

Costa Rica 2003

This is it. July 21st 2003 and I'm off to do something that I've thought about for 11 years. The company I hired for a trip to the airport was right on time.

Checked in and boarded the plane for Costa Rica by way of Havana, Cuba and San Salvador in El Salvador. I haven't been on a plane in a long time and I'd forgotten how much I love flying, but getting through airport security is a considerable pain. I can only assume it will get worse.

Havana was nice from what I saw through the planes window. We were not allowed off and only stopped there for dropping off and picking up passengers. El Salvador from the air looked fabulous with its lush jungle and volcanos dotting the landscape. Same deal though, never saw anything as we were only there to change planes and I never got out of the airport.

"...listening to Physical..."

Landing in San Jose was rather uneventful and I got off the plane, claimed my luggage, and was through customs in 15 minutes flat. I think other airports could learn something from this place. I also had to go through a metal detector and my luggage was x-rayed before leaving the airport. Asked for an explanation of the reasoning behind this, none was forthcoming.

Finally made it to the hotel in Playa Del Coco that I'd planned in advance at 7:00 last night. The total time to get here from my front door was 16 hours.

I ended up taking one bus and countless taxis to get from the San Jose airport to here. Near as I can tell so far, the taxis and buses almost always drop you off a little short of where you want to go. You end up taking just one more so you can get to where you wanted to go in the first place.

Oh well, it's been entertaining so far. You have not lived until you're on a Greyhound type bus for almost six hours with no restroom in the back. On top of that, you're careening through the Costa Rican countryside way too fast, listening to "Physical" by Olivia Newton John blasting on the bus stereo system. The song was half over before I realized what it was. I was too busy staring out the window watching jungle type foliage whipping by inches away at 80/100 kph. I actually started laughing out loud at how ridiculous this all was.

As I mentioned there's no restroom in the back. So every once in a while the driver would stop and one or two people would get off and relieve themselves on the right rear tire. I have no idea what these people did if more pressing matters needed to be taken care of. Don't know and don't want to know. How the women took care of all this, I really don't want to know. Other than that, my first impressions of Costa Rica? It's a beautiful country. Quiet, slow, laid back. Nobody's in the huge rush here the way they are back home, the driver of this bus being the exception mind you.

"...First thought? It's very salty..."

I talked with the owner of the hotel last night where I'm planning on starting and finishing my trip. I gave him minor details of what I want to do while I'm here. I'm going to give him the whole story tomorrow. My biggest problem, according to him? A 30 day water supply. That's a lot to carry in and he thinks it's a lousy idea to camp out on public beaches as there is always a certain undesirable element lurking about that will steal anything.

He suggested going to Santa Rosa National Park. I think it was a good thing I'd already checked it out. It has basic restroom facilities and a water supply, but he thinks it's contaminated, so I will have to take my own. No choice I guess. Now my general hesitation with this plan is what's the point in attempting to camp alone and suffering through 30 days of this when you're surrounded by other campers.

He says the camping season is over and it should be deserted as the roads leading into the park are pretty much impassible because it's the rainy season. Best bet to get there is by boat. So just maybe, I'll end up with a national park to myself. Well I doubt that, but this seems to be the only working plan that I have available.

I'm going into town today and check the boat option out and see if I can arrange something workable and reasonable. He told me it may cost around $60 to be dropped off and picked up. Let's wait and see.

I got up this morning at 5:30, walked over to the beach and swam around for a while. When I was in Venice Beach I only waded around a little, this was my first real swim in the Pacific Ocean. First thought? It's very salty.

"…a sawed-off shotgun hanging by his side…"

It was breakfast time at my hotel when I got back and I asked to speak to the owner Serge, and had a brief meeting with him for about a half hour. I decided to come clean and tell him exactly why I'm here, my intention to live off the land or starve trying. He probably thinks I'm nuts and he's probably right.

I met his daughter who has spent time in this park and she explained to me what to expect and the costs involved. She phoned the park to get some additional info for me and will talk to some friends about arranging a boat.

I have decided to go sometime on Thursday July 24th and if the time frames are right, I might cut my plan from 30 days to 28. I think I might need more recovery time than what I'd allowed myself. I think most addiction programs are 28 days anyways, aren't they? I seem to remember a movie called "28 Days" or was it called "28 Days Later?" The same subject matter I'm sure. I'll play it by ear.

Before paying a visit to the boat guys, I went to the local bank to get some Costa Rican currency. It seems when you pay taxis in U.S. dollars, you're always paying way too much. And, here I am trying to quit smoking and a pack of 20 cigarettes is app $1.25 US. How is this possible? I should start smuggling cigarettes from this country, I'd make a fortune. Well, maybe not.

It was interesting to walk into a bank with two guards and one of them is walking around with a sawed-off shotgun hanging by his side in one hand. Guess that's a pretty strong deterrent for any foolish notions. He was very nice though. He called me a cab when I was done. I was exceedingly polite and thanked him several times.

After the bank, I hit a grocery store and got a haircut. She did a pretty good job considering there was no communication at all. After that, I went to see the boat guys that had been recommended by Serge's daughter about a boat charter. They want $150 each way and paid up front. These guys are also telling me that well water is available and apart from stinking of sulphur, it's ok.

So some are saying it's contaminated, some say no. I guess I'll have to make a decision on taking my own or not, maybe a two liter a day supply. Not a lot, but sounds reasonable I think. That's one decision done, sort of. I'll have to shop around for another boat though, these guys are way too expensive. (I did check other charter companies, they are all the same and Serge's daughter never came up with any other options. Never saw her again actually.)

The next problem and this is a big one, is now I'm being told because it's a national park, fishing is prohibited. Anywhere! How can that possibly be right? This just put a serious crimp in my plans of living off the land. It seems that park boundaries extend into the ocean and roaming park rangers enforce this.

Depending on who you talk to, these rangers are hardly ever seen and you can fish if you are careful. Also, fires are allowed depending on the season and all trash taken in must be taken out. On the subject of fruit trees, most agree that they're there, you've just got to find them. So now what? Do I take the chance that some of this is correct and go with no food supplies or rethink this part? I don't think I can survive with nothing for 30 days and that was never my intention. I know I'm fat enough, but 30 days? Live off the land was my plan and I just wanted to get rid of all the junk and fast foods. So now I'm in a quandary. I'll make a decision on all this tomorrow.

"…chewed on by a 20 lb land shark…"

I went for a swim again this afternoon and walked on what I thought was the right path back to the hotel. Wrong! There were lots of stray dogs around and I had encountered them earlier in the day. This time however, one of them was more pissed off than in the morning and snuck up behind me and bit me on the leg. A good deep one. Drew blood.

I always thought about what type of creature could bite off certain body parts in the ocean. Never thought about getting chewed on by a 20 lb land shark. So now on top of everything else, I'm walking around wounded. I hope a bite mark is all I got from that damn mutt.

I've decided two things this morning. First I'm going to see a doctor about this dog bite. I'm not too worried about it, but several people here have made the suggestion of getting it looked at. Therefore, I called my gold-plated travel insurance company and they gave me the rundown on what to do. I pay the doctor and submit a claim later. I wonder how much a Costa Rican doctor makes. Anyway, I have an appointment with one in town at 4:30 pm.

The second thing is I will take a water supply with me just to be on the safe side, 60 liters for 30 days. It had better be enough. After my doctor visit, I'm going to go see those extremely expensive boat guys and make the final arrangements. I have no choice. Then I'm going to hit one of the cafes here and indulge on a big, fat, greasy meal. My last? Hope so.

The plan for tomorrow as it now stands is to check out of my hotel at 11:00 am and take a taxi to the grocery store to pick up what I previously mentioned. I'll make the final decision on the food part while I'm in there and then meet the boat guys at noon and I'm off.

"...No chance of rabies..."

I saw the doctor at 5:00 pm as he was running a little late. His office is on the ground floor of a garage, four chairs in a waiting room where normally your car would be parked. I found this most amusing and wished I'd brought my camera with me. Maybe I'll take a photo next time I pass by, that way my doctor can check out her office and maybe make some changes. Indoor parking. Hmmm. I'll run it by next time I see her. see what she thinks.

Anyway his name is Dr Alvaro Ampie Bermudez from Nicaragua, but I just called him Dr Alvaro. A very nice guy who apologized right off the bat about his English not being the best. I replied, which I've done about a thousand times by now, that my Spanish is just about as good as his English. Actually, if you're reading this, I think you've discovered my English ain't so hot either. We got along fine.

He asked me the usual background medical questions with the help of a Spanish/English dictionary. He feels there is little chance of me having rabies and prescribed antibiotics for the swelling. No chance of rabies? I wonder how he reached that conclusion. He also said that rabies symptoms may show up about 20 days after the initial bite. If that's the case I'll have been in the jungle (that's what I call it) 18 days by then.

I must say with being Canadian, I have never paid out of my pocket for a doctor before. More than anything I was quite interested in what a Costa Rican doctor charges. The set price is $30 with tipping being optional. Tipping? I did try and give him an extra $5, but he wouldn't take it. The cost of the prescription was $10 for 10 pills.

There were many jokes back at the hotel that night about what the boat guys would find when 30 days had passed. I felt so much better. All I thought about was Bob Barker and his famous line "have your pets spayed or neutered." Yikes again! Oh well, sorry to disappoint, but I had that done several years ago. Now I'm what I refer to as "female friendly."

After my visit with him, I went to see the boat guys. The final time frame is, leaving Thursday July 24th at noon, pick-up August 22nd at noon. I decided to do the whole 30 days. It sounds better than 28. Total cost? $300 plus a $20.00 credit card fee. There goes the budget! I was

14

told that for a price of $60, I would have to go with other people to share the cost and not at a time of my choosing. It was the best deal I could make and I was not happy. I also had to pay the entire amount in advance, which I positively did not want to do, but there's no way around it. These jokers better remember to pick me up or I'm screwed for sure.

"...my last supper..."

Went to a casino/restaurant and it had some of the most beautiful girls working there that I'd seen so far. I was thinking what a lovely souvenir one of them would be to bring home. All of them were decked out in the shortest black miniskirts I had ever seen. More like belts I'd say.

Oh, my last supper? A steak and baked potato with a ton of soda water. The soda water is another habit I'm planning on ending.

July 24th Day 1

Not much to say here except I'm packed, my minds focused on the ordeal ahead and I'm scared to death of what I'll find. Or not find. So as they say, "let's get it on."

"...and all he said was jump in..."

Got a taxi to the grocery store and bought 10 six-liter water jugs. I stared at the food sections long and hard, but decided to take my chances. Other than two apples left over from yesterday and 12 cigarettes left in a pack, that's it. 30 days rations.

From the store, I went and met the boat guys. They are a shifty looking bunch and I was hoping beyond hope that I had not made a huge mistake. The only one that I know a little from two previous meetings and who speaks reasonably good English is a guy named Wilber.

He and his pal loaded my camping gear and meager rations into the boat and I must say it didn't amount to much. Who said losing a few pounds and quitting smoking is easy. The lengths that I'll go to better myself. I wish I had some small amount of willpower like a normal person.

So into the boat I go. It was a 40-minute trip and had some beautiful scenery to look at. Hope I get to see it a second time on the way back.

We were there quicker than I would have liked and now the moment of truth has finally arrived. I cannot believe I'm doing this after 11 years of thinking about it. Wilber tied all the water jugs to a life preserver and tossed them overboard as well as all my camping gear. Now when we left, they brought the boat right up to shore, but because of the two to four foot waves here, they're staying about 300 feet offshore. Great! Wilber then decides to ask if I can swim. Now he asks? I replied that I do and all he said was "jump in and watch out for the propeller" as he disappeared over the side. Oh Boy! In I go and head for shore. That was pretty much the most exciting thing I'd done in a long time. Just shows how dull my life has become.

The campsite entrance was about 60 feet from shore and we gathered all my stuff up and lugged it in. With that, Wilber turned and walked away. I yelled at his back not to forget to come and get me on the 22nd. He turned, waved and mumbled something as he walked into the surf. I watched him swim back to the boat and they were gone. Man, talk about feeling total abandonment.

"…There is a beach!…"

I stood there with everything soaked and finally got a good look around and guess what? I am not alone! I'm not even close to being alone. This is the deserted park I read and was told about? Yah right!

I sat on a picnic table (a picnic table?) next to three Italians and they looked a little put out that I'm here. They're put out? Near as I can tell there are about a dozen or so people in here at least. I was told because it's the rainy season, the one road leading into this place would most likely be washed out. Not so! As I'm writing this, 14 newcomers just walked past me all equipped with tents and surfboards, all teenage surfers I think.

This plan of mine has been in the works on and off for 11 years and this is where I end up? It just goes to show what happens when you change your location. I know lots of about Tahiti and hardly anything about this place, so I guess it proves there's no such thing as too much research. I went from a totally deserted island in the

South Pacific to this? Hmmm.

The two park rangers I heard about just showed up in front of me. Remember the two guys that I'll run into a couple of times a week? They have a ranger station a few hundred feet from here. It's their home base and they sleep there. I find it incredible that nobody I had talked to prior to coming here had bothered to mention any of this.

Anyway, they speak no English and I speak no Spanish. I should have brought a translation dictionary, but considering I was supposed to be alone for 30 days, I didn't think I'd need one. They came for some cash, $6 admission and $2 per night, and one of them asked for one of my cigarettes. I'm down to 11 left. I could hardly say no and the faster they're gone, the better off I'll be. Get the no smoking phase of my plan started ASAP. Just imagine all the smokers, boozers, tokers, food and bikinis that surround me. Well, the last one I can handle. Maybe not.

Campfires are allowed this time of the year and there are fire pits everywhere and trash cans all over. I haven't seen any fruit trees yet though. I'm in trouble. Out of all the people I talked to and all the stories I heard about this place, they were right about one thing. There is a beach!

Day 2

"…The Edge of Seventeen…"

I did cheat a little as I said and had a few cigarettes left in a pack. Between the time I jumped overboard and the sun went down last night, my cigarettes are gone. I guess that makes me "Butt Free" so to speak. I'm sure I'll feel the effects soon, but what can I do, go to a store? Hardly. At least that part of my plan is working. So I'm officially a nonsmoker starting today. Let's see how long that lasts.

I met a couple of surfers camped close to me and they had seen me writing. So being naturally curious surfer types, they introduced themselves and asked what I'm doing here and what I'm writing. Well to say the least, after I told them why I was really here, they were stunned I'd set myself up to do this.

There were lots of handshakes and the word "Dude" was used most vigorously. I lost count. I guess I'm now a certified surfer dude, minus the board of course. Well, maybe a dieter dude would be more appropriate. Guess what? It started raining, does that a lot. I suppose it's because it's the rainy season. DUHH!

Things are looking up. I met one of the bikini girls from the group of 14 that I mentioned earlier. She was also curious about why I'm here. I explained once again and I get the feeling I'll be doing that a lot. Her big question was what I plan on doing for exercise. Hmmm. I thought just swimming around in the ocean five times a day would be enough. "No way," she said rather harshly. Turns out she's into yoga and I certainly would not have turned down a lesson or two. I asked her how old she is and she told me her birthday is next month. She'll be 17. All I could think about was some song called "The Edge of Seventeen." I retreated to my tent.

"...stumbling around the jungle stoned..."

It seems that pretty much everyone in this deserted place I picked knows about me already. The grapevine works quickly around here. Wish I could find a grapevine. My food problem is turning into a big one. I can't find any fruit trees anywhere and those ranger guys are always on the prowl, so fishing is out. I don't know what I'm going to do. The two surfers keep offering me tea and rice, their favorite food I suppose and I politely keep turning them down. At least I have to stick to the "no food but my own" rule and since I don't have any, it should be a pretty easy rule to stick to.

They called me over this afternoon as they were having a little party. I went over and was quickly offered the hash pipe that was being passed back and forth. I think I got enough problems to deal with and stumbling around the jungle stoned better not be one of them. Besides, all my life I've stayed away from drugs. I always told myself if I started smoking marijuana, I'd have a heroin needle stuck in me within 30 days. I know that's a massive exaggeration, but just that thought kept me out of the drug scene my entire life.

People like me with addictive personalities are best to steer clear of adding more addictions to the list. I retreated to my tent again. I get the feeling I'm going to spend a lot of time in there. I'm a loner in a jungle full of people. How is that possible?

Day 3

"…I'd rather smoke than eat…"

I can feel a bit of a routine starting in this place. Basically I go to sleep when the sun goes down and get up when the sun rises. By 9:00 am this morning two people have offered me three cigarettes. Of course, being as weak willed as I am, I took them. Maybe now you can understand why I wanted a place totally on my own.

I'm going to resign myself to the fact right now that while I'm not having a problem with the forced diet just yet, the smoking part is another matter entirely. Doesn't say much about me does it. that I'd rather smoke than eat.

If I can't truly quit though, then at least a major cutback is better than nothing. I'll just keep telling myself that. A lot! I'll have to keep a running tab on cigarette consumption just to see how bad I am.

Went out for my morning swim and brushed my teeth for the first time since July 24th. I just floated around out there and scrubbed them for ten minutes and rinsed in salt water. Tasty, and oh so clean and fresh.

The waves when they break are three to five feet high. That's my guess anyway and when they break lots of sand gets churned up. Sand, sand everywhere and there's no way to clean it up. It's in my clothes and all through the tent, but I am surprised it's not bothering me too much.

The bugs aren't as bad as I was lead to believe either. I'm here for 30 days, so what's the point of getting excited over stupid stuff. I must be getting old because this would normally drive me mad. Besides, I'm starving and I need a smoke. Sand and bugs are the least of my worries.

A guy here gave me half a pack of cigarettes. Guess he heard my plight. He just walked by with his backpack and tossed them to me. The cheating continues. Then a taxi that chanced coming down the alleged impassable road (remember that?) came to pick up my two surfer dude friends. A Taxi! What on earth are they doing here?

One of them whispered something to the cabbie and he came a-calling. He said he would pick me up a carton of smokes and bring them in on his next trip for $20. Guess what I said? Of course I said yes. What a weak-willed idiot I am.

Three hours later I spotted one of the surfer dudes walking around, so I asked him why he's still here. Seems their ride broke down a quarter mile down the road. The taxi driver called another taxi for help. Amazing! I think most likely my $20 is gone. because I never saw him again today. It's probably for the best anyway. I still need to make even a half-hearted attempt at quitting.

"...The Edge of Seventeen Part 2..."

I'd gathered a pile of firewood over the past couple of days and decided to fire it up so to speak. I'm not quite sure why, I don't have anything to cook on it. My suddenly forced diet isn't hitting me as hard as I thought it would, but my two apples are gone. I managed to make them last two days.

I got my comforting fire stoked up and my soon to be 17 year old surfer girlfriend stopped by. Turns out the group she's with are here for surfing lessons and the thrill of the camping experience. They're the group of 14 and not to be confused with the other surfer dudes I talked about. The tokers, remember? Gee, now I'm confused.

Big storm starting now, lots of thunder and lightning. Don't see these kinds of storms at home. Now back to the "Edge of Seventeen Part 2." She saw the pack of cigarettes that guy had given me lying on the table and wanted to know if she could have one.

"Smoking at your age?" I said. She's trying to quit, so she did the same thing I did, came here for however many days with no smokes. Well, that's not exactly what I did, but close enough. She said she's smoked for a year or so and wants to quit. A year? How hard can that be? I've smoked for 34 and I'm going out of my mind when I don't have any.

She asked how my forced diet is going and I told her I'm having no problem with it. I explained to her that I used to be a heavy drinker and had gone for long stretches before without eating. I told her that was my diet plan back then, all booze and no food. It worked real good too.

Most sane people use more conventional methods of dieting. I used straight whiskey.

Since I'm not supposed to give cigarettes to minors, I turned my back and played with my comforting fire for a few moments. Don't know what happened, but she was smiling. She said the group is being dumped into the jungle tonight alone with nothing but a sleeping bag each. Good luck with that one! Then the whole group will be gone in a day or two and there will be nothing good for me to look at. Oh well.

Day 4

"...lost 4 pounds and quit smoking for 20 hours..."

It rained all night and into the morning. I went for my usual swim and after just sat on the beach. I can't be getting bored already, can I? I've got 26 days left to go. Other than swimming, surfing and hiking there's absolutely nothing to do here. Since I don't and won't do the last two I mentioned, I'm going to have a problem I think. And don't forget I didn't bring a Walkman or a radio. No nothing, just this journal and four books. I suspect as the days trudge by, I'll be writing less and less in here. Oh, I finished the last of the cigarettes again last night, so I'm a nonsmoker once again. How many times is that now?

The taxi driver never came back so I guess I'm out $20. I kind of hope he doesn't come back. It would be the best thing for me at this point. I've been getting headaches over the last couple of days and I'm assuming it's because of the change in diet. Change to nothing! It also appears that I'm using a lot of exclamation points as this goes on! My irritability is starting to show up in my writing I guess.

Suppose that's to be expected. Isn't it!!!!

It's raining real hard now and some of the other campers are starting to pack up and head out. Maybe I should too, but how and go where? And what a colossal waste of money, energy and time this would end up as. "Be strong" I keep telling myself. This would still make a good book I think. "I lost 4 pounds and quit smoking for 20 hours." Bestseller that.

"…Do You Really Want to Say This …"

A guy I met at the hotel thought this would be the perfect opportunity to seriously look back on my life and how I feel about things and write them all down here. He's deep into spirituality and works with missionaries I think. That's not exactly my thing, but writing about how I feel? Well, I don't know about this.

I decided to give it a try and wrote many pages about my feelings on things and nameless people from my past. It was the most scathing stuff I've ever written or even thought of. With every page I wrote, I added on the opposite page in big letters, "Do You Really Want to Say This?" and had a huge arrow pointing to what I had written.

I guess I'll have to take a real hard look at what I've written and decide whether to leave it in or edit it out in the coming weeks. (I tore all those pages out and started fires with them about five days later. What I'd written was just too nasty, but I felt better having written it. I recommend that kind of therapy highly.)

Day 5

"...alone for a few hours anyways..."

Lots of thunder and lightning again last night and I didn't sleep much. I must have finally dozed off in the early morning though, because when I got up, everyone here was gone. I'm the only one here now. Part of my plan is finally coming together. I just wonder how long it'll last.

I took a quick walk around just to make sure I'm alone and except for the ever-present park rangers, I am. One of them said in broken English that he's going to find me a cigarette. One! WooooHoooo! How hard can that be when the other park ranger smokes? I almost told him not to bother as I ran out again last night and I'm not feeling so bad. But I'm weak-willed remember? If he brings it, I'll take it.

Went for a swim and when I came back more people are here. I'm really dying to see how awful this impassable road is. Oh well, I was alone for a few hours anyway.

But now to the interesting part, I almost called this section "Viva La France" and you'll understand why shortly. I went swimming again in the afternoon. I don't wear my glasses out there because they'll probably get knocked off and lost in the surf. I did develop the habit early on though, of constantly checking where I left my towel, only because I bury my valuables in a zip-lock bag below it. As I splashed around, I noticed two people sitting close by. I think it was two people or maybe just one large one. Remember no glasses on, so anything's possible. I'm going to stop here and start a new title.

"...Viva La France..."

Sorry, I had to use it. I've got to stop again for a second. I heard something behind me just now. When I turned around there was a three foot long iguana staring at me. It jumped up on the fire pit and stayed long enough for me to grab my camera and take a photo.

I'm just thankful it wasn't a 150 lb Jaguar. I would have lost 20 lbs the hard way. Anyway, this thing sat and stared at me for a while, then jumped back to the ground (flopped more like it) and waddled off. Back to the shadowy figure(s) on the beach.

I walked out of the surf and up towards where my towel and buried treasure was. I sat down and was drying myself when a man (I think), started walking toward me with a dark blob in his right hand. As the figure approached I put my glasses on and yes, it was a man holding a camera. He asked if I would take a picture of him and his girlfriend. Of course I said yes, if he would take a couple pictures for me.

As soon as I said yes, his girlfriend leaped up and ran over. Topless! All I thought was that there could be some benefits of not being totally alone. She grabbed the camera out of his hand and with her and I shoulder-to-shoulder, proceeded to give me instructions on its use. I wasn't paying much attention I'll admit. The thought of the girl being topless only lasted a minute or so then I kind of forgot about it. Strange, I must be getting old for sure! I spent about an hour with them and they were gone, so now this place is truly deserted again.

"...fat enough to live off myself..."

The park ranger I spoke about earlier stopped by with my promised cigarette. This one brings, I think, my total cigarette consumption since I've been here to 25. Only 25 in close to five days is really good for me, a major cutback. I usually smoke 25-35 a day. Even as I smoked it, I thought I could have lived without it. It's not my usual brand and don't taste so great.

This smoking situation can only get better over the next 25 days. Maybe I can actually kick the habit. The test will come when I'm back in the real world. The real world sucks. I'm starving. Don't know if I can do this for 25 more days. I figured I was fat enough to live off myself. I guess I was wrong.

Maybe I'll be able to wear my "Fat People are Hard to Kidnap" t-shirt soon. Can you believe I bought a t-shirt that says that and it doesn't fit? I'd ordered the wrong size.

Anyway, we sat and chatted as best we could. He asked if I could give him some English lessons. He's on duty here until August 10th. Of course I said yes as long as he gives me some Spanish lessons in return. He's just a young guy in 1st Year University and I imagine his memory of languages will be much better than mine.

I have come to the conclusion that I'm a complete idiot when it comes to learning another language. I just can't seem to retain anything. All I'm telling people I meet is that I have enough trouble with English, never mind Spanish. Doesn't say much for me.

He spotted something in the bush over my shoulder and just took off. This guy is always running around chasing animals. As I was staring at him running off, a crab walked over my foot. I almost fell off the picnic table. I'll to be a nervous wreck by the time I get out of here.

He came back and said he'd seen a falcon on the ground. He wants to be a biologist when he's finished school. That's why he works here. I'm tired.

"...shrunk to the size of a raison..."

My ranger friend came back around 1:00 pm while I was having a little siesta in my tent. He called out to me and I got up to find what? A plate of food! He said I look like I'm starving and maybe this will help me out. Seems I just can't win here. I resigned myself to the fact that I'm on a forced diet and now this. I certainly can't be rude to him (how's that for rationalizing this situation) because he thinks he's doing me a huge favor. I guess he is and I accepted it and actually tore right into it. It was chicken (I think) and beef (I think) and vegetables, rice and black beans on the side. He said it's called a "casado" and it's one of the main food dishes in this country.

It was honestly very good, but I think my stomach must have shrunk to the size of a raison (inside, not out) and I could not finish it all. Hmmm, who would have thought?

Between this meal and the one I had six days ago, I'm still waiting for this Montezuma's revenge I keep hearing about to set in, should be good for a few pounds off. More likely I'll be immune. I only ate local food and drank the tap water in my first three days in Costa Rica and what's happened? Nothing! I am "The Iron Man," for all the wrong reasons of course.

I cleaned up the dishes, but when he comes back, I'll have to tell him I can't accept any more food, at least not this week anyway. All of a sudden and who would have thought, my no smoking plan is working better than my diet plan.

Day 6

"...sucking on my dog-bite wound..."

I've changed my morning routine today. This swimming in the ocean business is not doing me a lot of good I think. I've used the shower facilities a couple times since I've been here, only once with soap. I thought the ocean would do an ok enough cleaning job and I left it at that. But it's like you're walking around with a film of some kind on you all day. Hence the routine change.

I had another open air shower of well water (one valve, one pipe) with lots of soap and the brushing of teeth, minus the salt water. Only problem was I'd kept my soap bar in a zip-lock bag and it's turned to mush. Now I got 24 days left and no soap. Great!

I think accidentally swallowing all that salt water isn't helping my diet either, so I'm considering admiring the ocean at a distance from now on. Besides, I'm getting a little tired of being pounded by the waves.

As I headed from the shower, I ran into my ranger pal. First question? "Are you hungry?" And I proceeded to explain once again why and what I'm doing here. Think I hurt his feelings, but I tried to be as polite as possible and I just can't take anything anymore if this is going to work.

I patted my big fat belly and said that with all this food he's going to give me, I'll end up "Mucho Grande." I think that was the correct term. He laughed, so I think I got my point across. Hope so! In the back of my mind though, I thought I'd just cut off everything once and for all. It's going to be tough going now.

I did finally get around to finding out what his name is only because he asked what mine is. At least I think he did. I'm not sure of the spelling, but I was positive he said it's

"Groberto." What kind of name is that? I'm not sure I'm spelling this, or anything else, right though. I wasn't, it's Roberto.

The bug problem here is not as bad as I was lead to believe, but these damn flies just will not stay off my legs and the sand fleas like sucking on my dog bite wound. Marvelous!

One pair of sweatpants cured that along with a pair of work socks. I must look quite the sight walking around like this. An Area51 T-shirt, sweatpants and socks with no shoes on and I haven't shaved since July 18th. Oh well, maybe people will leave me alone now or maybe I'll be mistaken for the park pervert. Great!

Another thing that's come up is I seem to be bruising very easily lately. Now that is clearly a bad sign. I take blood thinners because of a heart problem, and I'm supposed to get blood work done at least once every two weeks, more often if the blood levels are screwed up. So now I'm thinking that with all the changes I've made, diet and smoking-wise, I've screwed the levels up for sure.

There's no way to get anything done about it out here and I knew going into this that I could have a problem with this situation. I think maybe I'll cut back on that medication and hope for the best. By the time I get back, I won't have had a test done for seven weeks.

I don't know if I mentioned this yesterday, but I have company again. With all the campsites available here, they set up right beside me. Figures! I was proud of myself, sort of, as a couple of them were smokers and I didn't approach them to scrounge or buy one. I'm just too tired for all this. I want to be left alone.

The cigarette cravings are actually starting to lessen. The only problem is Roberto is on the prowl again to find me one. I guess I wasn't clear enough, but it would be a challenge to turn one down. I've got to quit these things once and for all.

"...right on my noggin..."

Something else I started doing yesterday is trying to keep the fire I have going 24 hrs a day. I know there isn't much point to it, but I need to keep busy and it keeps what bugs there are away. The fire I started yesterday did burn through the night so I'll keep at it. Even some of these rainstorms we've had don't seem to be bothering the fire. There's quite the canopy of trees covering everything.

I'll have to find out if this place is a jungle or a rainforest. I've been told it's classified as a dry forest. What the hell is that? It rains every day. At this point though, this is a rainforest as far as I'm concerned. Or maybe it's just plain "the edge of nowhere." I like the sound of that.

I'm also looking a little more closely at my surroundings and I think I'm going to move. There's a tree beside me now and if one of the main branches breaks off, it'll land right on my noggin. I'm bored anyway and it's time for a new view even if it is only 30 feet to the left.

Day 7

"...howler monkeys in the trees..."

I didn't sleep at all last night. Not sure why. Of course being up all night, I heard everything going on outside my tent walls. Between the trees creaking in the wind, the insects making an almost thunderous noise and what I think are howler monkeys in the trees, it was a long night.

Anyway, I got up tired as hell and reluctantly did my

morning routine and guess who showed up shortly after. The taxi driver I had given $20 to for a carton of cigarettes. I was hoping beyond hope that he either wasn't going to show or maybe now that he's here, he has a refund for me. Yah Right! The bag swinging from his right hand made that thought disappear real quick.

Sure enough he brought me not one carton, but two. Now what? I've been feeling pretty decent lately and now I'm faced going from having no cigarettes to having 400. This plan of mine is going from one catastrophe to another, but whose fault is that? Certainly not his, but why he brought two cartons is beyond me. Probably thinks he's doing me a favor. He does want an extra $20 for the favor though and he brought the cheapest cigarettes available here. They are rank and how do I argue with anyone out here? I don't and so without a choice, I paid him and sat down looking at my new smoke stash. So, do I keep them and have my no smoking plan literally go up in smoke? Hmm, what to do? I'll think about it, but I need to say something else right now. I'm not a happy camper.

"…6 days with only one meal…"

I've mentioned in here a couple of times already that this weight loss of mine is not working out exactly as I had planned. The only thing missing in this place is a "7-Eleven" store. I think if I'd been able to carry out what my original plan had been, the quitting smoking part would have been a no-brainer. Remove all temptation. No way of getting access to my bad habits. Remember me saying that? I can see and feel some difference in me as far as weight goes and I should damn well hope so. Six days with only one meal has to have an effect.

I am thinking now maybe doing this again next year.

Not that I'm giving up, but I'll just consider this a dry run. There's just way too much interference going on here. I'd obviously put this plan together much too quickly. Hard to believe, considering I spent 11 years on and off planning this, but this location was a last minute decision. I wanted to lose 60-75 lbs in total and always knew I couldn't do it here in one shot.

So I'm thinking that once and if I can ever pay this trip off, and that's a big if, I'll do this again and finish the job I started. I love Costa Rica, but I think next time I'll go where I wanted to in the first place, the South Pacific. Maybe do it with other people, people with the same problems as me. I wonder if there would be any volunteers. Maybe I could put a tour package together.

Actually, this type of thing would make a great reality television show. A bunch of people addicted to nasty stuff, stuck in the middle of nowhere with no access to their filthy habits, living off the land for a month. I should have tried that. Oh wait, I am. What day is this?

"...Alacran..."

Oh yah, it's day seven still. Anyway, later in the day I found myself surrounded by people again. Where the hell do they keep coming from? I go for a little siesta and I wake up in an amusement park. The rangers came by checking on things, no doubt to see if I'm still alive. Then some people that had camped near me came over. That makes five sitting at my picnic table with a huge language barrier happening. Their group is all from France. The French seem to love this place.

So here are five people that speak French, English and Spanish and can't communicate with each other. It was fun though, lots of hand gesturing.

Now I seem to attract all the animals around here for some reason. Maybe all they see is a big meal walking around here that's going to fall over any minute. So it was not surprising that Roberto found a scorpion under the table we were sitting at. He knocked it off and scooped it up in a clamshell. It's not very big, but I got a photo of it. Let's hope it turns out. I have my doubts about airport x-ray machines not affecting film exposed or not. We'll see.

One of the French guys ran to get his digital camera, took a couple of shots of it and I motioned for him take our little friend with him. If anyone's going to get stung, it'll be me, I'm sure. The Spanish name for scorpion is "Alacran" and even though it was only four inches or so long, the sting is similar to a bee. So they say! I don't want to find out.

"…pull out his gun and shoot me…"

Now back to my cigarette problem. I decided to give them to one of the ranger boys that smokes on the condition he gives me none back. I told him if I come begging for a cigarette to pull out his gun and shoot me. In broken English, he explained he has no gun. Another plan bites the dust.

Anyway, that's the best I can do, or maybe I'll just toss them in the fire and be done with the whole problem. I keep 400 cigarettes around me and I'll be worse off than when I got here. That's my solution and my story and I'm sticking to it. Besides, they are undoubtedly the WORST cigarettes I've ever smoked and even I won't smoke bad cigarettes.

Oh, did I mention that the French group and I are going with Roberto tonight to feed dead chickens to the crocodiles? Crocodiles!!! Where the hell did they come from? Apparently they hang around a lagoon that's only about a 1000 feet from here. That certainly is comforting news. I no doubt shall sleep soundly again tonight.

"...Is Your Name Shannon?..."

I went up to the ranger station in the late afternoon to drop off my smoke stash. As I was passing my cigarette treasure trove to him, he looked away and then nudged me. We were sitting on the deck of the station about four stairs high. I had my back to the railing and I turned to see what animal was approaching me now. I'm thinking all the time about that 150lb jaguar that I know is out there somewhere. And what really was approaching was an extremely attractive woman in a turquoise bikini, lugging a box of food.

Always the gentlemen, one of the ranger boys jumped up to assist her and relieve her of her burden. He beat me to it actually, but I was just too tired. Besides, it's not my job. They both walked into a ground level storage area beside the deck where all the campers store their food so the animals don't get at it. The animals never come sniffing around my tent at night. I wonder why. Anyway, they chatted for a while as she spoke perfect Spanish. When they were done, she walked out the door and he came back to take another look at his newfound smoke supply.

I was sitting on a stool and was going to give her maybe a ten foot head start before turning to take another peak at that turquoise bikini. I'm only human you know! Mind you, I don't look it at this moment. She walked out the door, made a U-turn and ended up standing right behind where I was sitting. She's on the ground, I'm up on the deck and she tapped me on the shoulder. I turned and was looking down at her when she said, "Is your name Shannon?"

I didn't say anything, as I was too stunned. All I could think was how she could possibly know that? After finally getting my voice back, I asked and it turns out she had met the "Surfer Dudes" in Liberia (the closest city) after they had left and they had told her all about me. What can I say except "my reputation precedes me?" Is that good?

We did spend some time together as she's here for two days with some friends. But in the time I spent with her, other than the turquoise bikini, I could not take my eyes off her's. She without a doubt had the longest natural eyelashes I'd ever seen on a woman. While she had several other natural attributes, those eyelashes were undoubtedly her most attractive feature. I'll be sorry to see her go.

Day 8

"…turning into an old woman out here…"

We went out to the crocodile lagoon around 7:30 last night. Roberto was armed with his two dead chickens and most of us had flashlights. That was the first time I had walked that far up the beach in total darkness and was pretty much the latest I'd been walking around since I got here. I'd forgotten how many stars there are at night with no city lights to drown them out.

We arrived at the lagoon, shining our lights in all directions and all you could see were eyes staring back at you. It was quite unnerving. Roberto threw the chickens in and the croc's just gobbled them up. It was quite impressive (if you're not a chicken), but I was glad to get out of there. I kept looking behind me just in case we were being attacked from the rear.

I'm turning into an old woman out here. I've never been so jumpy in my life and I'm starting to have a hard time focusing on what I'm doing. My mind is definitely starting to play tricks on me.

Today is basically the same routine and after another big storm last night, my fire is out and all the wood I collected is soaked. So much for keeping it lit all day and night. This will be my first day ONCE again smoke free and this time it had better last. I'm getting tired of writing about it and I'm sure you're getting tired of reading about it.

I'm supposed to take a picture of the ranger boys, but they stopped by way too early. I also haven't shaved since July 18th, three days before I left. I think I'm not looking so good and frankly I don't like it. It's all grey and grey is not my favorite color. I got a look at it in one of the car windows and the grey is another reminder that time is marching on. I'm going to let it go right to the end of my 30 days, might as well get the total bum look down pat. Maybe I should just leave it and go through Canada Customs looking like this. I don't think I'd get far though, I'm only a few hundred miles from the Columbian border and maybe Customs will get the wrong idea. I think it's time for some reading and sleeping. I'm fed up!

Day 9

"…the honey with the big eyelashes…"

Didn't sleep well last night, between the starvation diet and the nicotine withdrawal (once again), I'm feeling a little down. I think today I'll keep my mind off how I feel by fooling around with the sub-titles on these pieces. Amazing how a lot of this stuff makes sense isn't it? When

I go home and re-read this, I may have to change the last line to "actually makes no sense." Oh and I said goodbye to Katherine, the honey with the big eyelashes. I'm going to miss her. A lot!

One significant problem that has developed is trips to the park outhouse, or lack of them actually. The standing up part is working fine, it's the sit-down part that's ceased to function. I haven't had an outhouse sit-down since last Friday, eight days ago. That can't be good. I'm hoping it's the fault of the antibiotics that doctor prescribed me. If I remember right, don't they have a tendency to bind you up? I did use them up quite a while ago though. I'll let nature take its course.

I feel my mind starting to wander and I wonder how much of that will end up in here. I've got three weeks left to go and I'll most likely be a babbling idiot by the time I get out of here. Depending on who you ask, that could be said about me now.

I'm also wondering if I'm repeating myself in here. Fact is, I'm just too tired to go back over this and check. If I did, too bad! I am losing my mind after all. The heavens just opened up again. They don't call this the rainy season for nothing and I don't care what the technical category of this place is, as far as I'm concerned it's a rainforest. My fires out again and I'm soaked. I guess I'll be stuck in my 6' x 6' home for the rest of the day.

Day 10

"…I'll get my thumb ready…"

It was nice to get out of that tent, it's starting to feel like a prison. I'd pick this place over prison any day of course, except I need more supplies. Actually, any would be nice. What was I thinking?

The French people across from me are leaving today so I'm going to make my move. I was going to change locations a couple days ago, but I've been waiting for the French to clear out. That's got a ring to it.

I must have a half inch of sand on the floor of my tent. The only way to really clean it out is to pull all the stakes out, pick it up and shake the hell out of it. Oh and in case you didn't notice, I've knocked off ten days here already. Serge from the hotel I was at before coming here said I wouldn't last a week. Hah, who's the man!

I said the other day I tend to worry about things I probably shouldn't. Did I say that? The big thing that is really bothering me is what happens if those boat guys don't show up on Aug 22nd like they're supposed to. My mind is surely playing tricks on me and I don't know what to do about it. I'm worrying over this way too much and I put myself here. On purpose! It did seem like a good idea at home. Reality is a little different.

I'm surrounded by more surfers again. It seems this place fills up midweek and empties out on the weekend. I figured it would be the other way around.

I walked back from the showers this morning and talked to one guy who hitchhiked in and will do the same when he leaves. I'll get my thumb ready in case the worst happens. I'll have to clean up a little first though. Well, maybe a lot.

The time for moving is fast approaching and I'm feeling so alone, except for the fact I had a little lay down this morning and woke up to find I'm not. I'm really not. About 40 people just descended on my area. I looked out of my tent not knowing what's going on and where I sporadically have my fire going they just threw another grill on it and started cooking hotdogs.

I rushed out (I'm becoming territorial) and grabbed my corner spot at the picnic table I've been sitting at for the last ten days. I asked one of them who they are and why they're here. The one I asked actually spoke English and told me they're a bunch of university students on a day trip to check out the birds. Whoopee! They pretty much ignored me and then proceeded to put more food on the table than I'd seen in a long time, so much so that they dragged another table over.

I sat staring at two apples in a plastic bag one of the girls had and thought about offering her five bucks for one of them. I finally had to get out of there. Doesn't matter though, I'm moving to my new spot at 2:00 and the students are out of here at 3:00. I shall dream of hotdogs, tomatoes, apples and potato chips all night long.

"…just started beating erratically…"

I take a bunch of medication for an irregular heartbeat. In June of 2001, I had to go to the hospital and get "Zapped" as I call it. Basically what they do is wire you to one of those machines they use when your heart stops and zap, they shock your heart back to a normal rhythm. I've had it done three times since 1988 and I kind of like it actually. I figure it's as close to death as you can get without experiencing the real deal.

Anyway, I had it done then and it's been normal even since. TILL NOW! My heart just started beating erratically around 4:30 this afternoon. I took all the medication I'm supposed to take early and went for a lay down. I think what I'm doing here has been too big a shock to my system.

Day 11

Day 12

"...Can I stick it out for 18 more days?..."

Well as you can see, I was not feeling so hot yesterday. A couple of things happened, but I was too tired to write about them. The irregular heartbeat continues and this was the only thing I'd thought could blow this whole ridiculous plan of mine. I'm really caught between a rock and a hard place now. Do I continue what I'm doing or pack it in? The only way to fix this is in a hospital. A Costa Rican hospital? I don't think so.

Sometimes it goes back to normal on its own, but since I'm stuck out here I'm sure that won't happen. I've never really had a problem with this since June 2001 except for the occasional flare-up. This is the first serious reoccurrence since then.

I read over my travel insurance policy last night and it seems I'm covered for all this. I did buy the Gold-Plated insurance package, but I keep thinking back to 1988 when this all started. I basically walked around with an irregular heartbeat from 1988-2001. Can I stick this out for 18 more days? I'm not sure, but I'm going to try. It would be such a waste of time to quit this now.

You also need to remember that I weigh a lot more now than I did back then and I'm sure that's not helping. The worst side effect to this is it just saps your strength. Any moderate exertion and I'm done. I'm having trouble now walking a short distance without getting tired.

My new number one biggest fear is if those jokers (I shouldn't say that, but paranoia's setting in again) with the

41

boat actually do show up on Aug 22nd, I'll have to swim out to them. Meaning I'll have to fight through the surf to reach them and I'm not sure I'll have the strength to do it. I'm considering having them pick me up a day early so my time here will be cut back to 29 days to give me more recovery time. I should have cut it back to 28 days like I was thinking before.

Oh well, no point in second-guessing myself now. The question is how do I get a hold of them. I don't have the phone number and the ranger boys are reluctant to share their cell phones. Offer them money I guess, that always seems to work. I do have a number for Serge at the hotel I was staying at. Maybe I can get a hold of him and get him to call the boat boys. MAYBE, MAYBE, MAYBE! I'm tired.

"...felt a little sorry for me..."

Well, that's enough of that crap. I've decided to tough it out as best I can and that's that. I crawled out of my tent yesterday to find three people set up beside me. One's a girl from California by the name of Marshan. I've no idea if I spelled that right and with her were Matthew and Jane, her friends from England. I guess I wasn't looking to good and they asked me if I was ok. I explained my reasons for being here and they seemed quite surprised. Doesn't everybody?

Matthew felt a little sorry for me I guess and walked over with a big slice of pineapple and a half bag of the saltiest corn type chips I'd ever tasted. It was great and I made it last all day. They left shortly after. I crawled back into my tent.

Now today after ten days or so, I finally had to hit the outhouse for a sit-down. Three times! I'm feeling better by the minute. Well, not really. Anyway, I guess that's another problem solved. I solve one and two new ones crop up all the time it seems.

Time for a lay down and start reading my next book. This is, I think, my third day with no smoking. I feel so good! Not really.

Day 13

"...little piece, err, peace of mind I meant..."

Not much to say here. My heart's still jumping around and all it does when it's like that is make me tired. Food is on my mind right now. I'm thinking about the moment I walk back into my apartment on Aug 25th. What shall I eat first? Well, guess what? I dumped almost everything I had. I'd pay ten bucks for a single apple right about now. Hmmm, the price is climbing.

I was looking at my feet last night and they are in rough shape. The heels are cracked, with dirt and sand just jammed in there. Plus the nails on both my big toes have broken in half. I'm not sure why that happened.

Did I mention I stepped on one of those scorpions two days ago? I figured I was dead for sure, but the bottom of my foot just swelled up. It felt like a bee sting just like I was told, but since I've never been stung by a bee, it was a new experience for me. Yeah, the little snot got me good, but I got him good too. Now, back to my feet.

I go to a salon once in a while for a pedicure. Up to this point I haven't done much in the way of how I dress or what I look like. But for some reason, ugly cracked feet bother me a lot. Go figure. I remember that before finding out that I could get my feet cleaned up professionally, I tried to fix them myself. I went to the local hardware store and bought a palm sander. Figured I could do it myself. Wrong!

So now, the honey that does this for me tries her best to make mine pretty (what?) and to say she's attractive would be an understatement. She says she's been in some music videos, but won't tell me which ones and she's training to be a fitness instructor. I need personal training!

So while sleeping in my 6'x6' jail cell last night, I started dreaming about how bendable and flexible she must be. Now I don't usually remember what I dream about, but this one is burned into my memory. The next time she's sitting across from me, I won't be able to look at her in quite the same way.

Thanks for giving a 49-year old starving and nicotine stressed guy in the middle of nowhere a little piece, err, peace of mind I mean.

I went to sleep earlier than usual tonight as this place is filling up once again and I was hoping I could get that dream restarted. Dreaming never hurt anybody. Did it?

Day 14

"…I only have one match left…"

I guess I must be looking really rough now because just about everyone that camps here comes over to see if I'm ok. I wish they'd all just leave me alone. No more free food since the pineapple ring and bag of chips though. That's ok, I just have to tough this out as best I can.

I also seem to have underestimated my meager supplies. Because of my continued on and off smoking habit, I only have one match left. I guess I can scrounge one here and there to keep the fire going, which keeps going out because of the rain.

Also, I'm drinking more water than I thought I would and will probably run out before my times up here. The ranger boys have extra and they seem to give it out when people ask, but that doesn't mean anything. I'm sure if I run out there'll be a shortage all of a sudden. I don't think I can last till Aug 22nd. I'm feeling real bad and I'm tired. Real tired!

Day 15

"…He seems a little nuts anyway…"

I feel a little better today. I keep forgetting I'm in such a lousy mood because I haven't smoked in five days I think. I'm really starting to lose track of what I'm doing and when I did it, if I did it at all. I'm still worried about those boat guys showing up on the 22nd. I decided if they don't and if I have to, I'll walk out of here. OH YA!

I won't have much choice unless I can find a ride. I talked to the two people with the kids that are camped beside me. They hiked in and are going to hike it out. I can't believe they managed it with two small kids in tow and full camping equipment. It took them four hours. He seems a little nuts anyway and his wife doesn't seem too pleased about the whole situation. She had to carry the four year old the last half of the hike.

I figure if I actually have to hike it out of here, I'll pretty much abandon everything and just take the essentials. Oh, and the hike out is over 13 kilometers. I don't remember the last time I walked that distance and I can just imagine what kind of shape I'll be in 15 days from now. I'm thinking I'm deluding myself big time.

Day 16

"…The Curtain Falls…"

I met a couple from England last night out on the beach. He's on a cycling trip from Cancun, Mexico to Lima, Peru. He took a two week break to spend time with his girlfriend, who flew in from London.

We started talking about what they're doing here and I guess I was wobbling a little standing there and she was looking at me kind of funny. I pretty much told them what I was up to and how disappointed I was that most of the things I was told about this place were so wrong. No fishing anywhere. No fruit trees of any kind, least not around this area. I think she kind of suggested that maybe I should pack this idea in or maybe I did. I'm not sure. Anyway, we swapped more stories and parted company.

I ended up laying in my tent all night wondering why I'm doing this to myself. I had some pretty lofty goals in mind and I've fulfilled them, sort of. I've lasted 16 days here with hardly any supplies. There was no opportunity to try and live off the land, so to speak. I haven't smoked in six days, but I don't think I'm cured of that problem, not enough time has passed. The most important part of all is what do I do if these boat guys don't show up? You can see how much that weighs on my mind. I think about it constantly. I came here to make a point, I'm just not willing to kill myself trying to make it.

So, rather reluctantly, I have decided to bail out of this portion of my trip. I just can't deal with the almost total hunger, health problems and uncertainty of my ride out of here. So as they say in show biz, "The curtain falls."

"…how bad I'm feeling right now…"

I talked to the couple from England first thing this morning and they're going to give me a ride out. I'm very disappointed for two reasons.

One: That I couldn't tough this out for the entire 30 days.

Two: Even though I'd researched Costa Rica, because of such a short timeframe arranging this, obviously I didn't do a very good job.

I can't believe the planning and research that I put into this turned out to be so wrong in all the things I counted on the most.

I have decided to forgo the hotel scene and stick with tent life as much as possible. Actually, on that part I don't have much choice. There's no way I can afford to pay for hotels until Aug 25th. I think there is a camping facility close to where I was staying in Playa Del Coco, cost is $3 per night. I'm not too sure about this though. I guess I'll just try and carry on what I started, I'll just do it in a friendlier environment.

I still have the fishing equipment with me and maybe now I'll get a chance to use it. A couple of guys in the park that know I'm leaving offered me a box of cereal for my fishing gear. Ahhhhhh, No!

The couple that's driving me out is leaving at 3:30 pm, so I've got lots of time to pack up. I can't honestly describe how bad I'm feeling right now, both mentally and physically. I don't even want to write anything else. I'll pick this up tomorrow when I'm in Liberia.

Day 17

"...to be back to Civilization? Great..."

I woke up this morning looking and feeling lousy still and somewhat disoriented. Felt strange to wake up in a regular bed after all that time lying on a sleeping bag with clothes as a pillow. I have no clue how much weight I've lost, but I tried on my denim jacket and instead of the standard four inch gap, it overlaps two inches now. That's a good sign. I'll just need to watch what I'm doing as far as the food consumption goes.

Any number less than what I started out at weight-wise will be an improvement. I'm still a non-smoker though and that's been the toughest part of all. I've got the corner shops nearby again so I better steer clear. I guess I should catch up on what happened yesterday when I left.

Kristian and Gerri are the names of the couple that drove me out and we left around 3:30. This was my big chance to get a look at this supposed impassable road and I must admit it was pretty awful. Only way in and out of there is with two legs or four wheel drive. I found out the taxis in and out of this place are all four-wheelers. That explained much. The road was grim and took around an hour to go the 13 kilometers.

We passed several vehicles coming in as well as some people walking, all nuts, the lot of them, or maybe just much younger than me. We were in a Sidekick, which is not exactly my idea of reliable transport, but this thing actually handled the two foot mud-pits and the dry riverbeds. I was quite impressed. The scenery was fantastic driving out and with me in the back seat hanging out the open rear window, I got a magnificent view of where we'd been.

We hit the highway to Liberia and getting there was another half hour or so. Gerri asked me where I was planning on staying and I replied that I had no idea. I hadn't researched this out at all, shouldn't have been a need to. She had a travel guide, so I took a quick look through and picked the cheapest place. Found a hotel for five bucks a night. Perfect!

I told them to drop me off on the outskirts of town, but they drove me right to the front door of the hotel. I thanked them profusely and I hugged them both I think, I'm not sure. This place looked like a palace compared to where I had just come from. I checked in and got a lot of strange looks from everyone. I wonder why?

Into the room I went and just dumped all my stuff on the bed then went back to the front desk wanting to know where the closest restaurant was. Out the door I went, turned left, walked two blocks and there I was, in a Costa Rican Chinese restaurant. Amazing! Down I sat with more people staring at me. Do I look that bad? I'll check later. The waiter handed me a menu all in Spanish of course and before he could get away, I ordered. My order? #19. Didn't care what it was, I'll just take #19 and hope for the best. So I'm in a Costa Rican Chinese restaurant and what do I get? A big steak (I think), french fries (oh no), salad and a dessert. Looked great, but the only problem was I guess my stomach must have shrunk big time. No way could I finish all that. I knocked off maybe one third of it and left. So this is what it's like to be back in civilization? Back to the $5 Ritz and sleepy time.

"…decided to do something rather dumb…"

I got a look in an extremely small mirror in an extremely dingy bathroom this morning and "Oh Boy", not good at all. No wonder everyone is staring at me. I got directions to a grocery store and went there immediately. Bought some razor blades, which are needed desperately, as I had only brought some cheap disposables and there was no way they'd cut through the mess on my face.

Food wise, I just bought light stuff, fruit, vegetables and a plate. That's it! I did test myself though and stood in front of the shelves that have all my old and deadly favorites. I bought none. I feel that getting away from the terrible eating habits I had when I got here has helped me immensely.

I feel in my mind that maybe I've been able to sever the "I must have this" feelings that plague me constantly. I know at this moment I have no desire for the junk and fast foods. A definite good sign and I won't be ordering any more #19's while I'm here. That was an act of desperation and won't be repeated. So just maybe, the "get rid of the junk and fast foods" part of my plan worked. I guess time will tell.

I got back to the hotel and shaved that mess off my face. I cleaned myself up as best I could and went to talk to the hotel owner, Dennis, who speaks near perfect English. What a relief to hear that and I'm promising myself, I'm going to take Spanish lessons when I get home.

I decided to do something rather dumb on my first day back among the living. I asked Dennis if there are any movie theatres around here. I expected the answer to be no, but was told there is. He gave me directions and I jumped in a taxi.

Just imagine that yesterday I was sitting in a park starving and a little loopy around 2:30 in the afternoon. At 2:30 today I'm sitting in a modern and near empty movie complex in a teeny, tiny mall. And what am I watching?

"Charlie's Angels: Full Throttle." The change of venues over the course of 24 hours was mind-boggling. The movie wasn't so bad either. I went back to my $5 hotel after and crashed out.

Day 18

"…Sitting on a Park Bench…"

I think this is going to be a day of leisure here. It's Sunday so everything is pretty much closed. How's that song go? "Sitting on a Park Bench" and I guess that's what I'll do today. It'll give me a chance to catch up on some writing and think about what's coming next.

I did meet a couple today from Toronto, which is about 60 kilometers from where I live. It turns out they have a daughter that lives about one kilometer from me. Small world I suppose.

So seriously, I guess it's back to Playa Del Coco tomorrow for one final night in an upscale hotel. Serge has all my valuables locked up in his safe, so I've got to go back. Then its campsite hunting, but I'm going to wing it as far as that part goes, just wait and see what happens. If I can find an extremely cheap room, I might take that instead.

I've got 15 days left as of tomorrow and I started once again, seriously exercising as much as I can each morning. My strength is coming back, so I have no excuses. I had a couple of false starts in the exercise department, but it's time to knuckle down and do it.

One thing I've rediscovered over the last couple weeks is my love of swimming and I did it often. I'll continue that wherever I end up, it seems to be helping me weight-wise. I didn't do it much at home and the only reason being I was too self-conscious of my looks. That's the beauty of this place, you can do what you want and not care about it. If anyone doesn't like the way I look, so what, I'm never going to see them again anyway.

"...how much grief, pain and suffering..."

I finally got a close look at myself in a full-length mirror this morning with some good lighting. It appears I lost some amount of weight in the chest and stomach area, always a problem area for me. That's the spot I always seem to lose weight last. Middle age spread? Yah, spread all over. Oh well, it's a start.

My arms and legs have shrunk down also. I also lost a fair amount in my face and THAT'S got to be an improvement. My double chin is almost no more. Also, my skin has cleared up considerably, no doubt because of a serious shortage of sweet stuff. The lack of chocolate covered almond leaps to mine, only because I've gone 21 days without them. Figure a quarter pound of those a night (sad, but true) for I don't know how long, translates into lots I haven't eaten since I left. The result can only be a good one.

I'm going to start doing with my dangerous foods what I've done for a long time now with alcohol. I mentioned before I stood in front of the shelves of the grocery store and looked at all the things that are bad for me. I do the same thing with alcohol.

To this day when the opportunity presents itself, I'll stand in front of the section of a store with all the booze products and stare at them. I just feel the need to test myself. I'll just stand there with a bottle of whiskey in my hand, turn it over and around, and read everything on the label. All I think about is how much grief, pain and suffering this stuff caused me over the years. I've never left the store with any.

For an alcoholic, it's a very dangerous practice and I recommend it to no one, but it's just something I feel compelled to do. I wonder why it was so easy (so to speak) to stop that addiction, but so hard with the others. So I guess I'll do the same from now on with the foods that make me fat. Stare at them and think back.

I walked about six blocks out of the town center and back just looking around. I'm starting to understand the need to carry some water around, you start to feel a little faint after a while. Central America in August is just a tad warm.

I made it back to the restaurant I went to when I first arrived here and two bottles of water and a small bowl of noodles later, I'm feeling much better. Back to the $5 hotel and snooze time. Or so I thought. I ended up watching TV for a while. "Grease" in Spanish with no subtitles.

Day 19

"...Oh and the catch?..."

I'm packed and ready to hit the bus station. It's time to get my game plan going. I'm not sure how, but I'll figure something out when I get back to Playa Del Coco. I got to the bus station a half hour early, just so I could people watch a little.

Seems they're watching me instead, the taxi drivers I mean. First thing I'm faced with is a cabbie wanting to drive me direct from Liberia to Del Coco for $7.50. Now that's a 38 kilometer ride, so there's got to be a catch.

Well, it turns out the cabbies name is Manny from California and he speaks English of course. That was enough for me. It's been a while since I've had a conversation with someone in English who isn't a local. I took him up on his offer, although he pulled right into a gas station and asked for the cash then and there. The tank was a little dry so I gave him $10 and called it even. Oh and the catch? He steals passengers from bus stops along the way. Actually, I thought that this was a brilliant idea, although the jeep he was driving was packed solid by the time I got to where I was going.

Manny's favorite topic of conversation along the way? How many women have screwed him over in his lifetime. Man, his list was long and I started counting my list over in my head. Mine paled in comparison to his and I prefer to forget the lot of them. Mind you, one thing I've learned over the past few years is there are two sides to every story and I'm only hearing one of them.

I do think though I'll have to try and restart my so-called love life again. Other than a couple of meaningless relationships since March/2001, I've pretty much kept to myself. When you don't feel comfortable about the way you look, it kind of puts a crimp on things. But there's always time to find the next "Mrs. Ex" I guess.

"...Back Home, Sort Of..."

We arrived in Del Coco and Manny dropped me off at the hotel where I'd started my little adventure. I really like this place and wish I could stay here for the rest of my trip, financially though this isn't possible. I checked in and since Serge wasn't there, I grabbed a taxi back downtown. Surprisingly two things happened.

First, I ran into the head guy who runs the boat charter who was, of course, surprised to see me. He actually remembered my Aug 22nd pick up date at the park. That was the one thing that nearly drove me mad when I was camping. Would they remember to come and get me? I told you before I tend to worry about things I probably shouldn't. I gave him my tale of woe and he offers me a refund on the spot. Just like that. I guess I had these guys pegged all wrong. So I'll pick that up tomorrow at 11:00am.

Second thing is, I checked out the campsites close to here and they suck, so I went hunting for cheap rooms instead. I found a hole in the wall motel right on the beach for $10 a night. No more tents for me. My boat refund covers the motel cost for 12 nights and I got change left over for 12 day's worth of watermelons.

How best to describe the new digs? I would say a cross between staying in the Salvation Army (which I've done) and the YMCA (done that too). The only difference is the Sally Ann and the YMCA didn't have the Pacific Ocean 50 feet from my door.

"…I told you so…"

The next thing on my list? Waiting for Serge from the hotel to show up, so I can get all my personal belongings out of his safe. He finally showed up and was surprised to see me two weeks early. He repeated what he'd said to me before I left which was "I wouldn't last a week." Sort of an "I told you so."

I pointed out I lasted 16 days and of course got no comment on that. I gave him a general rundown on my ordeal and what I'd accomplished and failed at. I also told him I couldn't stay at his hotel because the budget is blown and I'd found much cheaper and dumpier digs down by the beach. I sure wish I could have stayed, but there was no way.

55

Day 20

"…shock therapy still seems to be working…"

The time has come to leave Villa Del Sol and move into my much less comfortable digs. Regrettable, but that blown budget keeps rearing its ugly head. I got my refund from the boat guys in full and walked over to my new home. It's very depressing where I am now after where I was, but it's got to be better than a campground. I just could not have faced another two weeks in a tent no matter what the reason.

I'm managing to keep the diet alive and the no smoking continues, but I can feel it's going to be a rough go. Best that I spend as much time alone as possible away from all the nasty influences. I did go to the grocery store to get some fruit and bottled water and once again tested myself while I was there. I stood in front of the shelves stocked with all my food and drink choices staring long and hard. I left with none.

My shock therapy still seems to be working. I was most pleased with myself. The soda water and chocolate called the loudest, but I resisted. I get the chance to resist again tomorrow. Must not fail now! If I give in, all this will have been for nothing. I'm trying to muster up the willpower I have stashed somewhere in my head to forget all this stuff. I'll try and stick with the sensible foods. I feel if I can keep the junk and fast foods out of my life, I'll be fine.

My 16 days of no food and few cigarettes seems to have given me the jump-start I needed. As I sit here now and think of those 16 days, I have to wonder if such drastic action was really necessary. What I know now however is a 30 day minimum food supply would have been my best bet. Oh well, live and learn.

Had a casado for dinner, it was the same thing my ranger friend gave me that day way back. It was very good and I'm wondering if I should just stick to one meal a day and fill up the rest of the day on fruits and raw veggies. Sounds like a plan I suppose and I'll play it by ear, like I do with just about everything else. There's a massive storm rolling in. I'm going to sit outside and get soaked.

Day 21

"...like a banquet of sorts..."

I got up early and had what is becoming my usual swim. I don't know what I am going to do when I get home without my own personal ocean. I'll have to think about that. The ocean is extremely convenient, but I miss Serge's pool already.

I have no food left here and this going to the store every day is becoming a pain. So I think I'll buy for two days and see if that works out. I have no access to a fridge or stove here, so I'll plan as best I can.

I walked over to the town square and grabbed a taxi and as always, I told him to meet me back at the store in a half hour. And as always, he never came back. They never do! All the taxis I've taken since day one and it's always the same story. From now on I not gonna pay them till I come back. This is the only complaint I have in this country. The taxis cannot be relied on. Even if I know the guy, it doesn't matter.

Anyway, back to my shopping spree. I bought some fruit and veggies again and that's all. No sodas. No dairy. No meat. No sweet stuff. After 16 days with zip, this is like a banquet of sorts. I haven't eaten such basic stuff in a long time and it's amazing how fast part of a lettuce, one tomato and half a cucumber can fill you up. The question is how long will this behavior last. I guess now it's up to me.

I have been told by the so-called experts it's better to eat like this several times a day than do what I normally do. I would starve myself all day and then pig out when I got home. I'd knock off whatever was available or I always shopped at the end of the day when I was weakest. Another extremely bad habit I'm told.

And let's not forget my beloved chocolate covered almonds. They were in the store today and I sailed right by them. It wasn't hard either. I guess I'm progressing, but again, time will tell. Especially when I get home. I'm sure that's what everyone will remind me of and actually, people are doing that now. "You get home and all the bad habits will come back. It won't last. It's different here." Hmmm, what can I say except they're probably right.

Let's not forget as far as alcohol consumption went, I was a loner drinker. I usually only drank in my apartment by myself. Very seldom I drank in public, so to speak. Two and a half years later I can sit alone in my apartment and there's no bottle of whiskey sitting in my freezer. I'm reprogramming my mind I suppose. Let's hope my brain doesn't have a meltdown.

Cigarettes are always in the back of my mind though, an extremely difficult habit to bust. Its noon, I'm tired. Time for a swim and a siesta.

Day 22

"...3 little red numbers..."

Didn't sleep much last night, some of the locals were out with the car stereos blasting a meter from my window. What can you do? I got up real early and hit the beach as the sun was coming up.

It was quite amazing to flounder around in the ocean doing nothing and watch this small fishing village come to life. All the tourists climbing into charter boats to go sightseeing, fishing, scuba diving and surfing. The surfers are going to where I was for 16 days. Do I envy them? Nope! I'm quite comfortable right here, thank you.

I'm trying to stay on my own as much as possible with no outside interference from anyone in my remaining days here of no smoking and big time dieting. The diet I'm on now seems to be working and I must say I'm feeling quite good.

At least that's what I keep telling myself. I'll know for sure when I step on those scales on Aug 26th at 3:00 am when I get home. It'll be interesting to see what those little red digital numbers have to say. In one way I can't wait, but at the same time I don't want to know. Success or failure of this entire mission depends on what three little red numbers say. Time for a salad, a big one. Mmmmmm.

Day 23

"...Happy Mother's Day..."

I'm succumbing to a serious food craving, pizza, and not the North American gooey and doughy slab of whatever's on it I'm used to. I can't help myself and it'll be the first one in a long while. I'll have to consider that my luxury food item. Just to be had on occasion.

I keep walking by one of the cafes here that make them in front of you with all natural ingredients and cook it in a kiln. I'm going to try it tonight. And yes I know, I said I'd stay away from that kind of thing, but old habits die hard and I'm doing my best. Besides, I am on holidays. Even I can only endure so much.

I am losing weight big time though and can see the results in the mirror. I think next time I get cravings, I'll just keep thinking about my clothes and what I see in the mirror. Can't hurt.

Also for what I think is the first time since I left on July 21st, I watched CNN English news. Seems there was a power outage in Ontario, Michigan and New York. New York City was the center of the story of course, with terrorism threats and all that. New Yorkers must be pretty jumpy and who can blame them. I've got to go there one day.

I took off this morning to get what I'm hoping is a final cash advance on my Visa card at the bank's ATM. My bank debit card doesn't work here, neither does my MasterCard, but I'm being told I can get a cash advance on my MasterCard through the grocery store, which I'll try on Monday. My Visa card's been on fire since I arrived here. It needs a rest.

Oh, and to all you mothers out there, "Happy Mother's Day" from Costa Rica. It's like a holiday here with almost everything closed. Great for moms, bad for me. Time to sort out my two day food supply and I took my clothes to a laundry here. All washed, dried and folded for $6.25. Is that good? I have no idea. But the girl doing it was cute (aren't they all) and I bought her a diet coke. That's almost the same as an engagement ring around here.

I starved myself all day (not really) in anticipation of my big treat of the night, that very spicy kiln cooked pizza. When I say spicy, WOW! It was the best, lightest tasting pizza I've ever had. Super thin and crispy. The cost was the same as getting the laundry done. I guess I'll starve the pizza off tomorrow. I must say I had 16 days of practice at starving myself. I'm getting pretty good at it. Bedtime for Bonzo.

Day 24

"...and get next to nothing in return..."

I thought about what I'm going to do for the next week sitting in Playa Del Coco. My options are limited, so I have decided rather rashly to grab a bus and go to Panama. I figured I'd stand there and stare into the canal. At least I can say I'd seen it. When sanity set back in, I decided to go back to Liberia for a night.

I've got to hit a real bank machine and find out what's going on with my personal bank account. Maybe I can get a cash withdrawal on my MasterCard there instead of waiting to try it at the grocery store on Monday. I think I explained before that these cards don't work in the local bank here. Besides no one at the grocery store speaks English. It's a hassle for sure. While I'm in Liberia, maybe I'll hit another movie or two. I'll make a real day of it.

I've also been giving a lot of thought about what I did here for 16 days with nothing but camping gear and a water supply. I mentioned before I'm thinking about doing this again with perhaps eight or nine other people and put my own tour together. I wonder if I need a license for that. Probably.

I can base it on 14 days in total with 10 days in the

park. I could put together an entire package including all the hotels and transportation and include all the meals before, during and after the park ordeal. I wonder if anyone would be interested in spending 14 days with me and not smoking or drinking and being on a forced diet for 10 of them. I could very well end up being the most hated tour guide in history.

And when you think about it, who better to put this together than me. I've done it once already and doing this several times a year would certainly strengthen my resolve in not smoking and avoiding all nasty foods. I wonder how many times I could do this without withering away to nothing. I sure would like to find out.

Next week when I get back from Liberia I'll research all this out and try and put a dollar figure on it. Think people with the same problems I have would be interested in this? This would end up being the opposite of an all-inclusive holiday. You pay big money and get next to nothing in return. Well, not really, but you get my point. Like I said, I'll put an all-inclusive 14 day package together and see what happens.

There might be some people who would like to try this, but would never, ever consider doing this on their own. No matter what happens though, I'm off to the South Pacific (we'll see) next summer for sure. Finish the job I started.

"…watching the pigeons pooping…"

The bus to Liberia just showed up. It cost .75 cents for a 38 kilometer ride. Not bad I guess. This is a beautiful country to see and you certainly can see a lot from a bus. I don't mind doing it at all. I arrived in Liberia and checked into the same hotel where I stayed last weekend recovering from my 16 day ordeal.

Then hit the bank and thankfully my debit card works as well as my MasterCard. Between them, I withdrew 42,000 colons (app $105 U.S) and hopefully that should get me through to the end. I grabbed a taxi and went to see a movie, but because of the time I got there, I only had a choice of seeing one with Tom Sizemore in it.

He's one of my favorite actors and what he was doing in this movie was beyond me. Maybe he needed the cash. I would have walked out, but I was the only one there and I figured the projectionist needed the work. I would have been better off sitting in the park watching pigeons pooping. The movie, funny enough was based on the same principle, minus the pigeons of course. If you've seen it, you'll know what I mean.

I had a quick dinner, hit an Internet cafe and headed back to the hotel. Back to Del Coco tomorrow.

Day 25

"…I'm a walking casualty…"

I caught the 9:30am bus back and its standing room only. The locals are off to the beach. It's Sunday and I guess even they take a day off now and then. As I suspected when I got back, the beaches are crowded. My luxury hotel suite is right on it, so I'm surrounded. Think I'll lay low till 4:30, that's when the first bus goes back to Liberia.

That's it I guess, my time here is running out and I think I've got an infection now in both ears. Too much salt water maybe, so I'll just stop getting my head wet. I try anyway. Hmmm. Dog bite, heart problem, scorpion sting, ear infection. I'm a walking casualty. What's next?

Day 26

"...can't go home empty handed, can I..."

I woke up tired and I'm not sure why, so I think I'll do absolutely nothing today. Maybe do some editing on what I've written so far. Good luck on that one. I did go down and talk to the taxi guys for a while. They're all complaining how slow it is and want to drive me somewhere. Anywhere! I declined and went to check out a couple of souvenir shops because that part of the trip is coming up. I can't go home empty handed, can I? I guess not.

I also worked a little on putting my 14 day tour idea together. I just asked around here about tent rentals and talked to the boat charter guys. There are no tent rentals available here, so that solves that problem. Maybe I'll check in San Jose when I get there on Aug 24th. That should work out real well because that's a Sunday. I guess that's enough work on this for today. Actually, I think it's time to scrap this idea. I just can't be bothered.

The weight seems to still be dropping, but nowhere near as fast as it did in the park. Well, that was to be expected and I've managed to keep the smoking urges in check. I still worry about re-entering the real world though. My world at home I mean. I was also thinking that four more days from today and I would have gotten my 30 days in. Oh well, next time.

Day 27

"...the edge of seventeen or turquoise bikini..."

I went to the Internet cafe here in Del Coco and checked up on my email and stuff. Time goes by so fast on a computer, except when you're writing a book and have no clue what you're doing. Two hours just flew by and it only cost $1.75 Not bad.

Today I have finally decided after a much worsening language barrier that I need to do something. I'm going to try and track down an English/Spanish dictionary somewhere. I'm not sure why I've been so stubborn about this, but enough is enough. Not let's see how smart I'm not.

Well, of course I went shopping for my two day food supply and what happens for the umpteenth time? Taxi drops me off, I specifically tell him to pick me up in a half hour, and he doesn't show up. And I know this guy, used him several times. I should have stuck to my new plan of not paying till I'm done.

However, to make a good situation out of a bad one, who do I run into? This guy comes out of the grocery store, looks at me with a big smile on his face and comes over with his hand outstretched. All I'm thinking is "who's this now?"

It was much more appealing when Katherine, the turquoise bikini girl introduced herself. Turns out he's the doctor who looked after my dog-bite, Dr Alvaro.

We shook hands and he could tell I had no idea who he was until he told me. See, 29 years of alcohol abuse does fuzz the mind up. He asked me how I was feeling, how the time in the park was and how the book is coming along.

I filled him in on everything and told him I'd written about my experience meeting him. I also told him that I wish I'd had a camera with me that day because I was taking pictures of the main people I've met on my trip. He seemed happy I'd included him in here and volunteered to meet me at 2:00 pm so we could do a photo together. Wish I'd gotten a picture of "the edge of seventeen" or "turquoise bikini."

Anyway back to Dr Alvaro. I made a deal with him. He checks both my ears for a possible infection at no charge and I'll send him a copy of this book as soon as it's done. He said he had no problem with that, so I'll see him at 2:00. AND! I guess I'll get weighed while I'm there and get the good or the bad news. Stand by!

Well I'm here and as far as the ear infection(s) go, this is the prognosis. I don't have an infection. I have wax build-up in my left ear and it needs to be cleaned out. I guess I'll wait till I see my doctor when I get back. She's scheduled for Aug 27th, I was thinking ahead. Now let's get on with the bad news.

The moment has arrived for the official weigh-in. I glanced around his examining room and guess what I don't see? A weigh scale. So I asked him the key question. "Do you have a scale to weigh your patients?" Answer? "No, I dropped it loading it into my car and I don't have the resources to replace it." I felt so bad for the guy that if I had the resources to buy him a new one, I would have. So that was that, no official weigh in.

So now I decided to ask him to get his stethoscope out and have a little listen to my heart, which he did. He knew I had a heart problem from our previous meeting and I could tell from the look on his face that the problem was back. I knew it for sure, but getting a professionals opinion doesn't hurt. So we lapsed into a very serious conversation, more him than me.

I've walked around with this on and off for 15 years, I'm used to it. He however isn't, and he wanted to personally put me into his car and drive me to the hospital in Liberia for further examination. Of course, I flatly refused because I know what a can of worms this will open.

He got pretty insistent about this even going as far as to explain to me what the consequences of this condition could be and his duty to me as a doctor to his patient, which as of now is officially me I guess. I again refused and tried to explain once again how long I've been walking around like this. I don't consider my problem life threatening, just a damn nuisance, and will wait till I get home and can see my own doctor.

"…what means cuter?…"

He finally accepted this, although he clearly was not happy with me. I still got the standard speech with the mandatory finger wagging in my face. I though back on how many times I'd had my doctors finger wagging in my face since I met her in 1995. I can't count that high.

I kept referring to my doctor as Dr Pam, which is what I always call her. Pamela is her first name, but Dr Alvaro was under the impression from the first time I'd met him till now that Dr Pam was perhaps a male Vietnamese doctor. How did the subject finally come about? Because I said I'd wait till I could see her because "Dr Pam is much cuter than you."

So after that was all sorted out we did a couple of photos and I promised him again that when all this is done, I'd send him a copy of this book. He's a great guy with a great sense of humor.

Day 28

Yesterday tired me out. I think all I'm going to do today is swim and sleep. Maybe I'll get my room lock fixed, I think it needs oiling. I can't get the key into the lock anymore, it's a little rusted from the salt water. Guess I should stop taking it into the ocean as I go floundering around. Duhhh!

Day 29

"…she said "what, you don't like sex?…"

Met my first Costa Rican hooker today. She'd spotted me swimming around by myself and cornered me when I came out. She must have known what room I was in because she positioned herself between the room and me. To make a long story short, she must have been in her late 40's and made me an offer I absolutely, positively could not refuse.

She was quite stunned when I did just that and the price plummeted. Finally, she said, "what, you don't like sex?" I replied "Sure, just not with you." I've had more than enough things happen to me since I've been here, I didn't want to push my luck, nor have to visit the doctor again. End of story.

I'm feeling a little down today because tomorrow would have been my 30 days completed in the park. I really feel like I failed in this whole thing. I just need better information and planning next time. And there will be a next time.

Day 30

I'm sitting here at 11:40 am looking at my watch tick off the minutes. At noon, the boat guys would have been coming for me. An hour later, I would have proved to myself that I could do this. I'm feeling like an absolute failure right now.

Saturday August 23rd

I called Serge at my favorite hotel this morning and am going over to see him. Besides, I left one of my denim jackets there. Why I brought jackets I'll never know. I don't feel like writing much today, I'm still bummed out about yesterday.

I guess I should add tomorrow's plans here though, because the bus ride back to San Jose will be a little bumpy and I'm having a hard enough time reading what I've written here anyway. Some of the stuff I've written in my journal is nothing more than a scrawl. So tomorrow, a final swim from 5:30 to 7:00 am, then cleanup and pack up, 7:30 check out and walk over to the bus stop and at 8:00am, I'm out of here. And I thought I felt bad yesterday. Reality is closing in all around me. I don't like it.

Sunday August 24th

"...white rabbit..."

It's time to leave the little sleepy fishing village of Playa Del Coco. Of course last night it wasn't so sleepy, it was Saturday night and some of the locals came out to blow off some steam. Car stereos blasting, yelling, motorcycles racing and cars driving by my window all night. Oh well, it's their village, not mine and it sounded just like home.

All in all, I had a good time here. I went out in the ocean at 5:00 am (I was early) and I still can't get use to the schools of small fish jumping out of the water a few feet from me.

Twice now I've been whacked in the head by large fish chasing small ones. This morning was third time lucky if you can call it that. A rather large fish jumped out of the water, hit my shoulder and slid down my right arm. I wish I was quicker, I would have had a free breakfast.

As I came back to the luxury hotel suite, there was a white rabbit in the laneway outside my door being chased by three chickens. This place is so surreal at times and where's the camera when you need it. Off to the bus stop and San Jose. Until next time.

"...overworked/underpriced hooker..."

The bus ride to San Jose was pretty much the same as on my first day, minus Olivia Newton John. I think this bus driver liked mucho silence and he didn't make the restroom stops I mentioned before, which was fine with me. I got to San Jose and went through the same crap as I always do with the taxis. They are a real pain, but I managed to get to a place I'd picked before I left Del Coco.

It's a hostel of some kind, age doesn't seem to matter and the price was right. Dorm rooms were $8, shared $11 and singles for $17. I called them yesterday to get some details, booked the $17 room and gave them my name. Of course when I got there, they'd never heard of me and the only thing available? The dorm rooms. Oh Great! So now I'm stuck in a room with three strangers.

Oh well, in less than 24 hrs I'll be on my way home and as always, I'm the oldest one here. What an honor at 49. All the youngsters looked at me like I should be in the Holiday Inn instead of here. Frankly that's not a bad idea and it's crossed my mind several times in the last hour, but to hell with it and them, I'm here now.

$8 is pretty cheap, but this had to be one of the worst places I've ever been in. Way too crowded and I don't belong here. "Tough it out" I keep telling myself. Think I'll grab another overpriced taxi into town and find a half-decent restaurant. Maybe I'll feel better.

Well, I was wrong. The taxi took me to a place where the food was just great, spiced to the max, my favorite. I walked around a little checking out downtown San Jose and ended up in what I would describe as a Costa Rican flea market. All the souvenirs I'd bought in Del Coco were half price here. I knew it! I was going to wait till I got here, but didn't want to chance it.

Ran into another overworked/underpriced hooker. I went back to the hostel alone. It was a shame they didn't allow guests. I'm sitting outside reading through this journal making some additions I'd forgotten about and corrections that are desperately needed. I need an editor for sure, but I think I'm it.

The skies just opened up again and I haven't seen it rain like this for a while. I'm hiding under a table umbrella and I ended up chatting with a guy named Jeff from Dallas until well after midnight.

Coincidentally, he's one of the guys I'm sharing a room with. We talked about many things and I filled him in on what I'd done in my time here. We discussed behaviors, learned and otherwise and how they affect people. He took some courses on this at North Texas University (I think) and seemed to know something on the subject. His feeling here is what I'd done wasn't too farfetched and if it works for me, who's to say otherwise. Well, of course I could not have agreed more. It kind of gave me some sort of validation that what I'd done wasn't too ridiculous.

"...SHE? What's this now..."

By the time we called it a night, I had elevated him from some guy who had taken a couple of classes in behavior sciences to a full "Professor of Behaviorology." He laughed, thanked me very much for the promotion and that was that.

I went back to my four person room wondering who else I'd be sharing with other than Jeff. There was nobody tucked in yet, I'm the first. Lights out and whoever shows up can stumble around in the dark. I'm tired, but I know I won't get any sleep here at all. I'll do it on the plane tomorrow.

I was there maybe two minutes and there's a key in the door already. The door opened and a figure walked it. Remember, I've got no glasses on, so I said to him in the darkness to turn the light on as I wasn't asleep anyway. She asks if I'm sure I don't mind. SHE? What's this now? She turned it on, took one look at me and asked who else is in here. I answered "there's another guy beside me and I have no idea who's above me." Imagine I'm 49 years old, sleeping in a bunk bed.

She looked around, grabbed something and walked out. 10 minutes later she's back. She says to me that she's moving somewhere else because she's not comfortable with this situation and obviously someone had made a mistake. She left. Good riddance, I wish I could have left too.

Monday Aug 25th

No sleep at all last night just as I predicted. The guy above me showed up around 2:00 am and was out of here at 6. I finally got up, had a shower, repacked and rechecked my bags and wrote this. Taxi at 11, flight at 1:50 and I'm outta here.

The Aftermath

I think I lost around or over 40 lbs in those 16 days in the rainforest/dryforest/jungle or whatever you'd like to call it. Not a very healthy way to do it, even I know that. I was 297 lbs when I left to do this, 266 lbs when I walked back through my door. So the final number after my 30 day attempt ended 14 days early was 31 lbs off.

I've actually managed to keep it off, the no smoking deal however died a month after I got back. It was just too hard to do both at once. The South Pacific is a pipe dream for me, I'll never get there so I've settled on as my second attempt...

Score: ½ successful on first attempt.

Newfoundland

"…I'm sure he was cheating…"

It's August 2nd 2004 and I'm going to try my weight loss program yet again. This time though, I'm headed to Newfoundland, a far cry from the Pacific Ocean I'll tell you. It's a Canadian province and island in Atlantic Canada. The only stop after Newfoundland is Ireland.

Flew out of Toronto via WestJet airlines, a company that tries a little harder. On WestJet, the flight crew isn't your regular uptight, get down to business type. The in-flight crew was very funny, especially Anne Marie, constantly cracking jokes over the intercom.

Any other airline would probably have fired her, but I think other airlines need their own version of Anne Marie. It was a very upbeat flight. She did her best Newfie accent when we landed. It was so awful.

Grabbed a taxi from the airport to a hostel I'd pre-booked in downtown St. Johns. I was met by the manager, Bill Furlong, welcomed in and I instantly changed his name to Bill Stressed. He was a real funny guy but doesn't want any stress in his life. He's not too successful at that I think.

The owner showed up later, Carola, and she was just as stressed and funny as Bill. I thought life was supposed to be laid back in Newfoundland. I'm only here one night, but it should be an interesting visit.

Played cribbage with Bill last night and managed a one/one tie. He's a self-professed crib champion, so a tie wasn't too bad. I was tired however, and I'm sure he was cheating. August 25th is the scheduled rematch. Anywhere else and you play best two out of three, but seems there's a different set of rules here. Whatever.

I was in St. Johns for a total of 11 hours and saw absolutely nothing of it. I'll have to fit in a sightseeing timeframe into my trip. Tomorrow I'm going to grab a bus from St. Johns to a place called Arnolds Cove. That should be a real leap into the great unknown. Arnolds Cove is where I start my 21 day self-imposed exile.

August 3rd

"...air out here is killing me..."

Woke up at 6:30 am and I'm off to the bus station. It's approximately 160 kilometers to Arnolds Cove. Was an entertaining ride and the scenery was fantastic. I got to the hotel I'd booked in advance called the Tanker Inn at 10:00 am and promptly went to sleep. The fresh and unpolluted air out here is killing me and how dumb does that sound. I guess my body isn't used to it.

Talked to the manager and explained to her what my plans are. I think having a finished book from my Costa Rican adventure is helping immensely. At least people I approach for help have an idea of what I'm up to.

She hooked me up with a fellow by the name of Melvin Newhook. I couldn't have been luckier. He owns the hardware store as well as the local bank. Bank? My eyes kinda went a little wide when I thought he owned a bank. What's he doing wasting his time on me if he owns a bank? Turns out he owns the building the bank is in. Close enough.

Melvin gave me a tour of Arnolds Cove and I let him pick a spot for me to sit for 21 days. The locals know the area better than me, so I put myself in his hands. Timeframe is to leave tomorrow 6:00 am. Melvin said we'd have to leave real early because of weather conditions.

Hurricane Alex hit North Carolina today and is swinging up towards us. If I get caught in the remnants of a hurricane, it should make for some excitement.

Had a nice dinner at the Tanker Inn. That will be it till Aug 24th, nothing but a fish diet for 21 days I hope! We'll see how good my fishing skills are with a $15 fishing rod. I have decided to try my luck at living off the land again. I know I'm taking a big chance, but I have a feeling it will work this time and I want to prove to myself I can do this. A fish a day will hopefully keep the doctor away. Spent the rest of my time watching T.V and sleeping.

Day 1

"…a fully equipped outhouse…"

Melvin called me at 6:20 am and said "we're good to go this morning." Quick shower, packed up and I'm ready by 7:00 am. We drove down to his boat, loaded up my once again meager supplies, which Melvin eyed with disapproval and slipped out of the harbor and into the fog.

I started to get that same sinking feeling I got in Costa Rica. "Why am I doing this" I thought once again. "Self-improvement you moron" was my answer once again.

According to him there are over 300 islands in this bay and I told him again to pick a spot he thought would be appropriate. We cruised around for a bit and he decided to drop me off on Sound Island. It's sparsely inhabited, so it's the best I can expect from the look of things.

On the way, Melvin caught a couple of fish, one for each of us. Dinner's not a problem today it would seem. Tomorrow however, will be another story. He dropped me off on a secluded beach where his brother has an abandoned cabin, which I'm told he never uses. Hence, it's abandoned.

I told Melvin this isn't exactly what I was looking for, tent life is what I'm after, not a cottage type deal. He just kinda gave me one of those looks, so I guess this is it. We got there and other than a small isolated cabin with no electricity, there's nothing around. Perfect! Sort of. If a massive storm hits, I can always break into the cabin for shelter. Not sure if my $40 Wal-Mart tent would stand up to hurricane remnants.

As we were pulling up to the shoreline, there was a caribou swimming across the channel going from island to island. Just some huge antlers and a head sticking out of the water. I got a picture of it as it came on shore just about the same time we did.

Got my first look at the cabin. It looks ok from the outside and there's even a fully equipped outhouse right beside it. The craftsmanship is unreal. 3 walls, half a roof, no door and no toilet seat. Paradise!

Melvin told me there's a trout pond nearby and waved his hand in the general direction of where it might be. Also, there's a large supply of bake apples around. Bake apples? What's that? He told me they are excellent to eat and expensive as hell to buy. I shall go on the hunt tomorrow. Don't forget, all I have with me at the moment is a fish!

Before leaving, Melvin said he'd check in on me a few times over the next three weeks. He doesn't like the idea of my lack of supplies other than bottled water.

The only thing in the back of my mind though was what cut my Costa Rican jungle trip short. Well, the old ticker is normal right now, let's hope it stays that way. Heart problems out here? Not good.

The tent is up next to the cabin so now it's time to make a fire pit. Lots of rocks and tons of firewood around,

I should be ok. Fire pit is done. I don't think I'd get a job as a stonemason or bricklayer though. Firewood is either damp or soaked. Also not good.

It appears the tail end of that hurricane that hit the U.S is really headed in this direction. That's what the news said this morning. Winds are picking up and it's getting cold out, maybe it's time for a little writing, reading and snoozing. Hope my fish is ok. I'll cook it up later.

I'm up, actually got a fire going and cooked that fish. I have no butter, oil, salt, pepper, nothing. Maybe I should think these things through more. I did bring a small grill from an old barbecue, at least that did the job. I just tried out my cell phone by calling my home number and surprise, surprise, it works. Think I'll order a pizza. That's it, bedtime.

Day 2

Well, the hurricane leftovers never materialized and it rained last night for about 30 seconds. Was thinking about swimming today, but the water is cold!! Definitely not Pacific Ocean temps. I'll try my hand at fishing today.

Melvin said there's a trail behind the cabin (I don't see it) and if I walk it about 15 minutes, (straight up) I'll come across these alleged trout ponds. I think I'll save that excursion for tomorrow. Suns out, it's pretty hot today and everything is drying up. Good!

Day 3

"...I'll go caribou hunting instead..."

Last night had quite the gale (is that what you call it?) and I thought for sure the tent was coming down or blowing away. Only thing holding it in place was me. I set up pretty close to the water's edge on day one and it was six feet away from me last night. Maybe I'd better move the tent back a little. I'll go survey the damage and then head off into the woods. I gotta find these trout ponds and all these fruit bushes and trees I was told about.

This is only day three and I'm fed up already. Not a good sign. Everybody I talked to before coming here about fishing from the shoreline just hummed and hawed. That means what? Yes, I'll catch something or not? I'm getting the feeling the answer is the latter. I did try the fishing deal on the shoreline till it got dark last night and nada, nothing! Maybe it's the cheap fishing gear or maybe it's the operator. ME! 18 days left. OMG! All I've had in three days is one fish.

The first time I did this with no food, it was "exciting and new." Now, not so much. A boat would be handy right about now. Oh well, if this fishing doesn't work out maybe I'll go caribou hunting instead. There are tracks on the beach right past my tent. Hunt with what? Only thing I can shoot it with is my camera. Maybe I should concentrate on these trout ponds and fruit trees.

I hiked all the way to the top of this island and guess what I found? Nothing! Lots and lots of blackflies and that's it. I followed some sort of rainwater run-off ditch/trench all the way up. Guess that's the trail. I think I'm in trouble. This is Costa Rica all over again.

I got back from my little hike and what's 50 feet from my tent? Another caribou! Tried fishing on the shoreline for two hours and nothing. Back on the starvation diet again. Trust me, they don't seem to work. Guess I'll go read.

Day 4
"...FEED ME!..."

Last night was very eerie, it was so dead calm. There were no sounds at all. Usually when the insects shut up, you know something's going on. The night before I thought the tent was going to be pulled right out of the ground, the wind was so strong. Last night nothing. Even the water was flat, not a ripple. First the wind kept me awake, now the silence is. I'm wondering how much I've slept since I've been here. My feeling is, not much.

Stomach is trying to tell me something though. FEED ME! Tried fishing again last night and right now it's only 7:00 am so I'll give it another go. My concern now though is this is not the right spot, maybe I should pack up and go somewhere else. Should I sit here and try and tough it out 17 more days or go try out camping in more hospitable places. But where and how do I get there? I don't know what to do. It was never my intention in Costa Rica to starve myself for 16 days and it's not my intention to do it here. Once was enough!

It's raining here again and foggy. The fog just continuously rolls in and out. I fired up the cell phone and I think I left two messages for Melvin. Not sure. My cell is working, I can hear the greeting on his machine, just not sure if my messages are being received. Guess I'll have to wait and see.

It's raining real hard now and the wind has picked way up, so I've decided to break in the cabin beside me. My first Newfie criminal act. This thing is abandoned but locked up tight. Maybe there's some food in there. More motivation!

Well, getting in wasn't so difficult after all, one of the windows was open a half inch. I found an old rotting wood ladder in the bush and used that to get in. And what do you think I found? The whole place was like a laboratory experiment in mold gone wild. Mold absolutely everywhere! It was climbing the walls, all over the ceiling, even on the kitchen table. It looked like someone had packed up real quick and left, never to return.

I'm no mold expert, but I swear I could taste it in the air and you don't have to be an expert to know that's a bad thing. There were beer bottles on the table, cigarette butts still in the ashtray.

I found a box of canned food on the side of a bed and took a quick look through it. The tops and bottoms of the cans were corroded with I don't know what. There were black spots on them. More mold? Only thing I found that appeared to be salvageable was one can of baked beans.

I opened them with a knife I found, took one sniff and tossed them to one side. So that's that. I spent a grand total of five minutes in there and had to get out. I'll bet you thought I was going to eat the beans didn't you? Nah, I'm not that desperate. Not yet. I think day four is done.

Day 5

"...was I stranded?..."

Another fierce wind and rainstorm last night, I had to go out around 2:00 am and re-stake the tent down. I sat here most of the night thinking what my options are now. I have 16 days left and it would appear no real food supply.

I forgot to add yesterday that I was standing on shore as a boat went by. I didn't wave him down. He just looked in my direction, slowed down, turned around and came to within 20 feet of me. He asked me the big question "was I stranded?" I said it was starting to look that way. Asked him if he was heading for Arnolds Cove with the answer being "no."

I explained that I had left messages with the fellow that had dropped me off here and if he didn't make an appearance by tomorrow morning, I will consider myself stranded and start flagging any passing boats down. He said he'd check in with me in a day or two and see what's up. Funny thing was he never asked what I was actually doing here.

Back to the "no food supply." I've tried the onshore fishing deal with no success. I've gone up and down the shoreline trying different spots. Nothing! So I think that idea isn't going to work. I thought about this last night and came up with two options.

Option One: Get the hell out of here any way I can and chalk this up to experience once again and move on. Move on to where? I have no clue. It's the only sensible thing I came up with since I don't have the funds to stay in St. Johns for an unexpected two weeks. I'll have to take a flight out of here earlier and that's it.

Option Two: If my buddy Melvin ever shows up, maybe he can take me back to Arnolds Cove and I can stock up properly for the 16 days I have left. I'll pay for the extra trip back and forth. It has to be cheaper than staying in St. Johns for an extra two weeks. Obviously my grand plan for living off the land is a grand illusion, for me anyway with my limited "survivor" skills. (There's that word again!) If I had a proper food supply, 16 days might be doable.

The weather is harsh and I'm sleeping on the ground, but that, surprisingly doesn't bother me. The lack of a food supply, that's what's screwing my head up.

So that's my two options. One other thing though. It's pretty hard to keep a fire going in the constant rain and dampness here. Those caribou walking around are starting to look tasty again.

So that's it I guess. I cleaned up the area, its 9:27 am and there's nothing to do the rest of the day. I'll go read something and this day is done. If anything exciting happens I'll add it here. If not, tomorrow I start flagging boats down and give them a real compelling tale of woe.

Did a quick run through of the cabin again. Popped open another couple of tins of food and everything is spoiled. That's it! Tomorrow I start flagging boats down. I've had enough of this!

Well, shock of shocks, Melvin just showed up. He never got any of my messages and he stopped by to give me a tub of worms. I explained to him the fishing isn't working out here and I couldn't find the trout ponds or fruit trees or bushes. He waved his arms around randomly telling me they are "up there." I thanked him for the worms, but told him he has a passenger instead. I've had enough of this nonsense.

He had one of his grandkids with him and was going to pick up a bunch more. "No problem" I told him, but either way, I'm outta here. I gave him a tour of the moldy cabin and he figured it was best to burn it down. Agreed!

Melvin gave me a ride to a town called Swift Current which had a store and a phone. He took off to do whatever with the grandkids and told me he'd pick me up in three hours. I bought some drinks and food at Monk's

Place and called the Tanker Inn to reserve a room. So it looks like that's it then. My camping experience in Newfoundland is over. To hell with Option Two, I'm done here!

August 9th

"…Dildo…"

Got back to the Tanker Inn hotel around 8:00 pm last night, ate and crashed. Had all my clothes washed, changed my flight to this Wednesday, and was on the bus back to St. John's this morning.

I can't believe how utterly gorgeous this province is. If I could have, I'd have taken a bus ride from one end to the other, stunningly beautiful here. And the names of the towns around here are equally stunning. Somebody had sex on their mind big time when these names were thought up. Town names like Dildo, Conception Bay, Blow Me Down, Come By Chance, Happy Adventure, Heart's Desire and Tickle Cove. Shall I go on? Nah, you can look these up if you don't believe me.

I managed to get back in the place I was when I first got here. They were booked up, but Mr. Stressed found a spot for me. It's only till Wednesday afternoon. I can't believe how drained and tired I am. Maybe I'm getting too old for this nonsense.

August 10th

I finally got to see the city of St. Johns before I leave. It is very beautiful. Kind of reminds me of San Francisco. The streets are all on hills. The houses are the same, all angled at their base. It must be horrible here in the winter dealing with driving up these streets.

I went up to Signal Hill where in 1901, Guglielmo Marconi received the first successful transatlantic radio communication. And later on I took a whale watching tour. Saw lots of whales right next to the boat. The weirdest part of the tour was at the beginning. We were pulling out of the harbor and I sat in the back on the right side, leaning on the railing. All of a sudden, the boat ground to a halt, groaning and creaking as it did. I thought we'd hit a sandbar or something. Then all this grey muck went past on the surface of the water.

After a minute or so, the engines revved up and off we went. I asked one of the crew what we had hit. She looked at me kind of puzzled and said we didn't hit anything. Hmmm. So I asked her why we had stopped. She replied, "Oh, to scatter the ashes of some woman's husband." What!!! Well that explained the grey muck. Only in Newfoundland.

Aftermath

Well, that whole trip was a failure weight loss wise. I walked through my door, weighed myself and had actually put four lbs on. Now I'm back up to 270. GOD! I'll have to try something else.

I looked up Sound Island on Google Earth and there are bodies of water on the top of the island. I didn't realize the island was that big and I didn't see them from my vantage point. Either way, Newfoundland is beautiful. Go for a visit there if you can.

Score: Still only a ½ for 2 attempts.

Vancouver

I did this trip over Christmas and New Years in 2004/05 more on a whim than anything else. Not much planning went into this one. Mind you, the same can be said for the previous trips. A flight, hostel, hotel and ferry planned out in advance, that's it. I just needed to get away and the warmest place in Canada at this time was the Vancouver, British Colombia area. By warmest, I mean not below freezing. I didn't have the funds to go anywhere else. So here goes another desperation trip into the unknown with me weighing in at 275 lbs when I left.

Dec 16th

Left Toronto at 7:30 am, arrived in Vancouver at 9:35 am. That was quick. Love those time zones. I stayed at the Cambie hostel in downtown Vancouver only because of its proximity to the Fast Lynx harbor ferry. My plan was to take the ferry to Nanaimo and then onto Tofino, my final destination.

I chose the Cambie hostel because they offer free airport pickup. Of course, I called and there was no driver available. Probably there is no driver. A taxi was going to cost $24 so I took a bus instead. Cost on that was $3 and I had to transfer four times. One hour later I'm at the hostel. No driver. Hah!!!

I'm tired as hell and crashed out immediately. When I woke up I went down to the common room which all hostels usually have. They have a T.V, couch and what not. I met people from Germany, Australia, and Japan. Very exciting. Yawn. In all honesty, my hearts not in this. Why am I doing this!!!

Dec 17th

"…Island Dick…"

Went to bed early last night, up at 5:30 am and walked around the foggy deserted streets a bit. Came back to the Cambie, checked out and walked over to the ferry terminal at 8:00 am and I'm off to Vancouver Island.

The "fast" Lynx ferry crapped out ten minutes into its run. A piece of driftwood I'm told got stuck in the water intakes. We got going again a half hour later. There was a mini bus waiting for 11 of us because the ferry was late. 11 people jammed together for a two hour ride. The driver made the Costa Rican bus driver from 2003 look like he was standing still.

The ride from Nanaimo to Tofino was unreal. Rain, rain, rain and I and the others thought he was going to flip the bus over. Racing around hairpin turns and tight curves. Signs said slow to 50 km, he slowed to 90. Everybody inside the bus had that look of "this is it." Never been bounced around, up and down, back and forth so much in my life. When I got to the hotel, called "The Whalers on the Point Guesthouse" I was physically burned out. Checked in and straight to bed, quaking under the covers. Very, very scary ride.

Got up and spent the rest of the day trying to make arrangements for camping out either in the Tofino area, Vargas Island or Hot Springs cove. See, I did actually do a little advance planning.

Called one guy recommended to me named "Island Dick." He's the equivalent of Melvin from Newfoundland. And old Dickey boy flatly refused to help me arrange anything. "If I'm going alone" he said, he won't help me. Hmm, firm believer in the buddy system I guess. I called a golf course with a primitive campground. All I ever got was an answering machine. Don't look good so far.

Dec 18th

"…lions and tigers and bears, oh my…"

Thought about this all night and this morning and maybe I'll have to forget this whole plan. Can't get any help from nobody! Then, I walked down to the dock and found a floatplane sightseeing service. Toby, the woman I talked to was extremely helpful, although as with everyone else, thinks I'm nuts.

I made arrangements with her, weather permitting, to fly to Vargas Island tomorrow, cost is $60. She gave me more details than anyone else so far on what the camping setup is there as well as who's around. There's an escape out of there by water taxi if things go horribly wrong. How I'd get a hold of them wasn't explained. Cougars, bears and wolves in the area could be construed as horribly wrong, right? Reminds me of "The Wizard of Oz" song, "lions and tigers and bears, oh my."

I'll take a walk up to the grocery store today and start putting together a 17 day supply list. No more taking people at their word that I can live "off the land" no problem. I've heard that twice now and had nothing but problems. Mind you, absolutely nobody is telling me to go into a deserted provincial park in Dec/Jan with nothing. There is a guaranteed water source there so I'll take only a couple of six liter water jugs with me. Only downside to this is it's always overcast and raining here so far.

Day 1

"…bikini clad beauties…"

Well, the floatplane is a go for 1:00 pm. Checked out of the hotel and slugged everything over to the floatplane office. They took care of everything. It's the pilot, me and two others in a four seater floatplane. I've never taken off from the water before. It was very exciting. The view was spectacular and we were there in 15 minutes. Saw a bunch of bikini clad beauties at the hot springs area, as we were landing.

We pulled up to the dock, where a guy named Sean has a huge boat docked alongside, which he operates as a Bed & Breakfast. Maybe I should stay in that. I hauled all my gear to the campsite, took one look at the ground and realized the tent idea is a no go. The ground is like a mud pit from the rain.

Luckily for me there is a tool/storage shed right beside where I was planning to camp. Broke into that and now I have a dry, unheated shelter with a set of bare wood bunk beds. Damn, it's cold and damp here.

Started raining as soon as the plane flew off. My winter parka and all the clothes I'm wearing are soaked through. Big problem I see is things are not gonna dry out here. Put all my other clothes on and hung up the wet ones inside the shed. Waste of time though, nothing's going to dry in this climate. Well, at least it's not snowing like the rest of Canada.

Very cold night, glad I brought a cheap air mattress with me. Will have to work on getting a fire going tomorrow. Outside of course.

Day 2

"…I'm stunned!..."

Worked on getting a fire going till 2:00 pm. Lots of chopped wood around here and I tried many times to start a fire with what I considered to be "dry pieces." That was an absolute waste of time. Someone very kindly left a full size axe here. I started chopping big pieces into smaller ones, hoping the interior of the wood might be dry. That actually worked. Tied a rain tarp I have with me high over the fire to keep the rain off. Hope I don't melt it. I hung my wet clothes next to the fire and they are actually drying out. Woohoo! Success!

I'm getting cold again, I need that winter parka dried out for sure to wear in bed tonight. Must be 0 degrees Celsius or maybe even a little lower at night. No rain today, big surprise. Went through my food inventory, looks adequate. Found the water supply hand pump. I have no idea if it works or if it's frozen up.

On checking out my supplies, I found that I forgotten to bring candles. I'm always forgetting those damn things. Also could have used some rubber boots, it's a quagmire here.

There actually is a water taxi that goes back and forth to Tofino every day. I'm stunned! Some actual factual information that's true! Maybe I'll grab that tomorrow and stock up on the things I stupidly didn't bring, the aforementioned candles and boots being number one and two on the list. Clothes are dry unbelievably and it's time for bed.

Day 3

"...Straight to the laundromat..."

Woke up cold as always. Time to properly restock. Went down to the dock and waited for this water taxi, a no show of course. I went back to my tool shed and double checked what I'm short of, because one way or another, I need certain items to survive out here.

As luck would have it, the float plane showed up at 10:00 am dropping people off to go to the hot springs. I made it down to the dock before he left and grabbed him. He was a different guy than the one I had on Sunday, but he knew about me. Hmmm. I told him I needed a ride back to Tofino to restock.

I think he thought I was quitting, and admittedly that did cross my mind, which is why other than my video camera and wallet, I left everything else behind. That way I have to come back. 15 minutes later, we're back in Tofino.

I hit the store and bought some rubber boots, a proper hat, gloves and a bunch of candles, which is what I'm writing this by right now. Also, grabbed three tins of barbecue lighter fluid (woods too wet), more bottled water and some more cans of food. And I recharged my video camera, which is a waste of time I think as all that happens when I pull it out is the lens fogs over because of the cold and dampness.

Straight to the laundromat and I stripped off practically everything I was wearing and tossed it all into a dryer. One jacket, four t-shirts, one sweatshirt, two pairs of sweatpants and three pairs of socks. Everything I'd brought with me on this trip, I was wearing. Quick stop at a restaurant, had a sandwich and three cups of tea and back to the plane. All this done in less than two hours.

Arron, the pilot was on a mail run, so I got to see much more than my initial flight in. Absolutely gorgeous country, must look fabulous in the summer. Back to the dock, back to my "hut," sweating and heart racing.(oh no) I collapsed on the lower bunk and after laying there for a bit, started wondering where all the steam was coming from. It was coming off of me. From my head, through my t-shirt and my sweatpants. For someone with the health concerns I have, this body still works pretty good, considering the abuse I've put it through over the years.

From all the steam coming off me, I must have a lot of internal heat. Is that good? I'll have to ask the ladies, if there were any around of course. Once again, I'm alone and it's for the duration I guess. 14 more days. Oh God!

Played with the fire and had a chocolate bar. I bought three. One for today, one for Xmas, one for New Years Eve. Pretty exciting huh?

Day 4

"...Quite pitiful indeed..."

Was nice to read all night with my newly acquired candle lighting system. Best $15 I ever spent. It's early in the morning here and very cold. The cold woke me up. Tried sleeping without the jacket on, a bad idea.

Dogs are barking across the channel, there's a small First Nations village over there. Will try and get the fire going at first light, yes is still dark out. It's damp, damp, damp. Everything always feels so damp.

Surprisingly there's been no rain the last couple of days, but the sun doesn't beat down where I am. Too much tree cover. I forgot a watch so I'm using my video camera clock. Damn. its 7:27 am Dec 22nd 2004. It truly feels and looks like its 2:00 am outside. Still dark, cold, no noise except for the aforementioned dogs. Oh wait, just heard a duck quacking, my day is complete. 7:57 am now. Time flows a little different here. Slow, like molasses!

Gonna try and shoot some video today, I haven't shot one frame. Kinda hard when the lens is always fogged over. Slept most of the afternoon. The sun is setting now and the First Nations village across the channel has a rock concert happening. Tribal drum music I mean. Sounds pretty cool actually. I hope I don't start dancing around my fire. Pitiful looking fire anyway. A few sticks of soggy wood in the lid of a barbecue I found. Quite pitiful indeed.

I asked Arron the pilot yesterday if there was any chance of catching fish by the shoreline. I brought my equipment from the Newfoundland debacle. He said no, but I should try anyway. He figures it would give the members of the village across the channel a big laugh though. Now THAT'S a confidence builder if I ever heard one. Night time and its cold, cold, cold. 13 days left. Oh my!

Day 5

"…two armfuls of dry wood…"

Around 4:00 pm I had a visitor. His name is Ike, from the First Nation village across the channel and he was just looking around. Most likely wondering what my deal is. He said rustic cabins are going to be built right where I am, maybe four or five. No more tents for people if they don't want to use them. My timing is as always, just a little off. Mind you, a tool shed is pretty rustic.

Anyway, he took a look at my pitiful attempt of fire building and pronounced that "the wood is too wet." No kidding Sherlock! He disappeared for five minutes and came back with two armfuls of dry wood. Where the heck did he find that? I asked. Just a wry smile in return.

Within two minutes he had a roaring fire going. WOW! He said he'd come back on the 26th to check up on me and wanted to know if I wanted him to bring me back anything. Let's see. A load of that dry wood? A television? A satellite dish? A kerosene heater? A generator? I thanked him and politely declined. What a dummy I am. Ike however is my new best friend.

Day 6

"...I am the crypt keeper!..."

Hmm. Xmas eve today. Where should I really be? Maybe I'll do this again next Xmas & New Years, only somewhere warmer and with supplies. After three attempts at this, I think I have all the kinks worked out. And people say I'm a slow learner. Hah!

Fire building today much easier with dry wood. Everything Ike brought yesterday I put in my crypt. That's my new name for my tool shed. I am the crypt keeper! Gonna decorate for the holiday I think. A sprig of fir tree decorated with my dry socks and empty tin cans. Now how much more Christmassy can one be?

Think I'll read the rest of the day and night away. I brought a book written by Doyle Brunson, the poker whiz. Maybe I'll actually learn something useful.

Day 7

Well, it's finally here. "Joy to The World" and all that bunk. I'm not a big Xmas fan, so being here is not so terrible. I'm going to do nothing today. It's raining hard, so I'll spend the day in my crypt. That's all!

Day 8

My fire is back to where it was a couple of days ago. All damp. I keep adding that barbecue light fluid on it, but that's not working either. An older woman walked down the path to where I am. No idea where she came from and I didn't bother asking. We talked for five minutes, then she was gone.

Temp here getting down near 0 degrees or below. I'll have to sleep tonight with all clothes on again. Geeez, I look like the Michelin man with all this on. Tomorrow I'm past the halfway point of this "adventure." Nine days down and eight to go. Can't quit now, I'd like to though. Hey, that rhythms.

Day 9

Got the fire going first try. It's a clear sunny day at least. Had my one can of peaches this morning, that's it for the day. Oh, Ike never showed up yesterday with my pizza. Did I ask him for one? Starting to feel my focus and attention drift.

Day 10

Woke up this morning near frozen. Must have been below freezing last night as there is ice on the mud pits. My feet are numb and I can feel it progressing up my legs. I think it's time to pack this in. I've had enough! I've lost some weight, don't know how much and don't really care right now.

I packed up what little I had and trudged down to the dock as Arron was due soon on his regular run. Man, my feet are killing me. What's up with that? Oh, I put my nice rubber boots on the wrong feet. If that's not a clue to bail, I don't know what is.

Arron showed up on schedule, I explained to him what's going on and he just said "hop in." Didn't have to ask me twice!

Made it back to hostel and unfortunately, they don't have any private rooms available. The one I had last time is occupied, so I have to take a shared dorm room. Great! More bunk beds.

First things first, I washed all my clothes and then headed for the showers. Man, I look grim. I actually had people staring at me. Showered and shaved, I look back to normal. Now it's time to formulate a plan B. I certainly don't want to hang around here for another week, so a quick call to the airline and I'm outta here. I'll leave tomorrow, same route, same ferry and hopefully not the same bus driver.

Going back was a repeat of getting there. Stayed at the Cambie hostel overnight and they actually gave me the free ride to the airport the next day that I never got when I arrived here. That's all folks.

Aftermath

That's three attempts in a row I had to bail early. Not a good sign for my master plan. Not good at all. I did weigh in at 270 when I got back. God!!! I'm wasting my time. Money too!!!!!! If you want to check out the bed and breakfast that was docked on Vargas Island where I was, it's called the Innchanter. I should have stayed there.

Score: Still ½ for 3 attempts. Damn!!

Antigua

"...drug smugglers..."

Landed in St. John, Antigua at 3:30 pm on Dec 18th 2006. When I got off the plane, there were I was told, some big name dignitaries in attendance. Surely not for me, I thought. That was definitely wishful thinking. They had a steel drum band playing, balloons everywhere, even T.V cameras there to record the event. What event? Well Delta Airlines had just landed their first plane here. Woohoo! Party!!!!

After all the hullaballoo, I grabbed a cab to the Cappuccino Hotel. I'd arranged this in advance, first and last night. I met Beverly, the owner, who was very nice and very pregnant, eight months along. The hotel wasn't high class, but a nice place for the money, $50 a night. Antigua is more expensive than what I'm used to.

All the stores were closed because it was a holiday of some kind. Maybe they proclaimed a national holiday just for Delta. Managed to buy two cans of soda and one bottle of water from a barber shop. Talked to the owner and filled him in on my plans here and asked him if he knew anybody with a boat for hire.

Next thing I know I'm in his car off to see a friend of his with a boat. One hour later I'm making a deal with his pal to take me somewhere up the coast to a deserted beach he knows of. He'll drop me off on Dec 20th and pick me back up on Jan 14th. $100 bucks each way. The $200 total included a trip up the coast tomorrow to check out some sites (that never happened) and he'd come once and check up on me sometime in my 25 days there. A little pricey I thought, but what can you do. So I landed here at 3:30 and had a done deal by 6 pm. Not bad in 2 ½ hours.

He did tell me about a deserted island near here, but warned me that drug smugglers use it as a drop-off/pick-up transhipment point. He said it was up to me if I wanted to go there. I declined.

My barber pal took me back to the hotel and I still don't have any food as everything is shut down. All I brought with me was a small container of raisons. Guess I start my diet sooner than expected. Watched a Law & Order SVU marathon the rest of the night. Night has fallen here and the bird and insect noise here is incredible, and I'm in the middle of a city. Reminds me of the Costa Rican rainforest.

Dec 19th

Pretty uneventful day. It's my one day of downtime as I don't leave till tomorrow. Thank God the stores are finally open. I checked out the supermarket for supplies I'm going to take and the price of everything. Bought some stuff to get through today.

Met up with George the boat guy later in the afternoon to finalize our deal. Price dropped to $75 each way as the little tour today had been scrubbed. I also found the local casino. Lost $20 and left. That's why I don't gamble much. My feeling always is every time I put a quarter in a slot machine, I shall never see it again. Back to hotel and watched television all night.

Day 1

"…nude beach…"

Well, it's that time once again. A leap into the unknown and once again, I put my trust in a total stranger. One day this will backfire on me I'm sure. Let's hope this isn't that day. Checked out of the hotel at 11:30 am and off to the docks.

George was right on time (a good sign) and I loaded my two bags into the boat and went to the market to pick up 25 days worth of supplies. In case you're wondering, I always keep the important stuff with me at all times, passport, cash, etc.

I bought what I though was a decent amount of supplies that would last 25 days. Bottled water, canned goods and 3 boxes of raison bran. Gonna have to eat that stuff dry. All loaded up and off we go.

Antigua has a beautiful coastline with many beaches and resorts. The last beach we passed was the only legal nude beach in Antigua. Think I'll stay away from that one. Swung around a point jutting into the ocean and there's my home for the next 25 days. Stunningly beautiful! George picked this because the beach is 90% submerged rock, which I'm assuming is the reason this beach is deserted. We landed on the 10% that wasn't.

George jumped out from the front of the boat and I stepped over the side and promptly disappeared under the water. He didn't mention the shoreline drops off rather suddenly. Felt my glasses get sucked right off my face as I went under. Never did find them, good thing I had a spare set. Anyway, that was my first swim in the Caribbean, never been here before.

We unloaded everything and George is ready to leave.

I paid him and reminded him my pickup date is Jan 14th. He just grunted, gunned the engine and he was gone. That's not particularly encouraging!

Now I finally have what I've been looking for, a deserted tropical beach all of my own. Set up my tent under a large thorn bush, arranged my supplies, everything's good to go, now what? Maybe I'll chase down the three little pigs that just walked out of the bush. Wild pigs I'm assuming or else the owner can't be far behind. Wouldn't that be a kicker if he dropped me off next to a pig farm? So, maybe bacon for breakfast? Ham and eggs? Oh wait, no chickens spotted yet. No frying pan either.

It's getting late, the sun is setting into the Caribbean. How idyllic and romantic and I'm here alone. While pondering that, I fell asleep.

Day 2

"...We eyeballed each other..."

Interesting night last night. I only slept a little. I was kept awake most of the night by all the sounds around me. Wind, surf, insects and grunting pigs among other things. After a while I couldn't separate sounds real or imagined. Like, I'm sure I heard music last night. Maybe it came from an offshore boat or the nudist beach I passed yesterday. It's not that far away. The only thing separating me from them is the bluff on my right jutting out 400 feet into the Caribbean. There's no shoreline to walk around it and it's pretty steep, on my side anyway.

I'm trying to picture all these nudists dancing to that music. Must be law against that. If there isn't there should be. Oh well, to each his (or her) own.

Woke up this morning to a tent full of sand, going to

be a full time job keeping that under control. Helicopters fly over constantly, four or five yesterday, four today so far. I also seem to be in the flight path of jets coming and going. Lots of noise here.

It's so nice to be alone. Had a family of seven anchor about 75 feet offshore this afternoon, five kids, two adults. I left my tent, which can't be seen from the water and walked over to the high point of the shoreline. The kids spotted me first and there was lots of fingers pointing. Dad was snorkeling and the kids swam ashore. We eyeballed each other, but never spoke. Dad finally saw me, called the kids back, packed up and left. Am I that scary? Time for my sunset swim.

Day 3

"...you trying to kill me?..."

Last night I could hear someone talking and a dog barking. I took a look out the tent flap and in the moonlight, sure enough, they were at the end of the high bluff on my right. I could clearly see the silhouette of a man and his dog. I have no clue where they came from. He kept throwing a stick over the bluff and the dog would run to the edge of the bluff and look down, then back at him possibly thinking "you trying to kill me?"

Got my first coconut today. I was lying beside one of only two coconut trees on this entire beach, which, I'm guessing could be half mile long end to end. Anyway, how I'm going to open it is another matter entirely. Bash it with a rock I guess.

On that bluff to my right, there are maybe a dozen goats grazing. They belong to the guy with the dog? He own the pigs too? No idea.

Two kayakers just rowed across the bay. They started to row in, saw me and changed direction. More visitors just arrived on the other end of the beach. For a deserted place, this place is pretty busy. three guys in a boat came ashore, two disappeared into the bush with two boxes on their shoulders while one hung back looking in my direction as well as scanning the area. OhOh! The two came back, minus the boxes and they all jumped in their boat and cruised the shoreline right up to where I was sitting. They looked at me, I waved at them and they left. You can come to your own conclusion of what they were doing. I did!

Day 4

The two kayakers from yesterday are back today, they came ashore about halfway down the beach from me. I didn't approach them and they did the same. They're on holidays I guess and want to do their thing just like I am.

I got that coconut open. Peeled the green stuff off and used a tent stake and a rock to put a hole in it. Tastes ok I guess. An acquired taste I'm thinking. Busted it open with the rock and gave the white stuff inside a try. Very tasty.

Goats or sheep or something are bleating behind me on the bluff somewhere. I'll have to start practicing my spear chucking. Lamb chops for dinner. Mmmm!

Day 5

Not much to report today. Had some more of that coconut. Took a walk on an extremely wide path today about 30 feet away from me. If I didn't know any better, I'd swear a tornado cleared this path out. More likely its hurricane damage though. There's uprooted trees all over and boulders where they shouldn't be. Gonna take a long walk up there in the coming days and see where this path goes. There's what looks like a half dried up lake on the right of the path. Oh ya! Its Xmas eve!

Day 6

"...She proceeded to get topless..."

Merry Xmas!! Woohoo!! Wow, four exclamation points almost in a row. I'm getting excited over nothing. Went looking for more coconuts, no luck. Lots in the trees, but I'm not climbing them.

Spent most of my day getting the sand out of my tent and clothes and trying to get a sand flea infestation under control. They are having a feast on me! Finally broke out the insect repellant and sprayed everything. Looks like I've got the measles with all the bites.

A boat anchored offshore late this afternoon with a man and a woman on board. She proceeded to get topless. A very nice show. He got bottomless. Shows over.

As I was sleeping last night, I was awoken with very loud snorting that sounded like it was two feet from my head. I sat immediately upright and thought "grizzly bear!" After two seconds, I remembered where I was and dismissed that idea. It's pitch black out, no moonlight or stars out because of cloud cover. I slowly unzipped the inside tent flap and there was a horse eating a half apple I'd tossed out the tent that night. Bad idea I suppose.

He stopped eating it, sensing I was there and brought his nose to within six inches of my face. Only thing separating us was tent screening. I could feel his breath on my face. This thing tame or wild? I have no clue. Also, I'm assuming it was a he.

Horses and pigs and goats, oh my! That "Wizard of Oz" line comes in very handy. All I'm thinking is what's next? Of course as we all know, the deadliest animal walks on two feet and my mind drifted back to the guys with the boxes at the end of the beach. No trouble with them yet!

Day 7

"...$250,000 a week..."

Started raining early a.m. That did in my plan for the big walk down the "tornado" path I mentioned earlier. Guess it's me and Jackie Collins for the day.

Took a quick swim and two guys showed up in a Zodiac boat. We said hi to each other (first people I've talked to since Dec 20th) and they walked around checking the beach out. They jumped back in their boat, waved and took off. Hmm, what's that about?

An hour later two different guys show up, same boat with folding tables in it. I helped unload them and asked what was going on? Turns out there's a private yacht coming with a crew of 12 and 10 guests on board and they're going to have a beach party here. Seems I'm the fly in the ointment, because this place is supposed to be deserted. I told them I won't bother them, I'm here for some alone time myself.

This big-ass yacht came into view and anchored in my bay. My bay! More crew came onshore setting up giant umbrellas, tables, chairs, and coolers full of yummy stuff I'm sure. I'd asked one of the crew guys who these people are and was told they are "big shot New York investment bankers." Damn, and here I was hoping for Britney Spears to show up.

They brought the big shots over who water-skied, jetskied, went snorkeling, ate and drank large. Everything that, I found out, a $250,000 a week yacht rental can provide. I got here for $75 bucks! And guess what that gets you? Hopefully, picked up again.

They finally packed up and left. Ho-hum, time for my 5 star dinner. Dry raison bran and a banana.

Day 8

"…who the one guy is that doesn't fit in…"

Went out for a morning swim and what do "I spy with my little eye?" A Zodiac boat headed my way again. Same crew guys came onshore so I went over and asked them what's going on again? Seems the yacht guests loved it here so much yesterday, they want to spend another day here. Well, that's just wonderful! I suppose if you're spending 250 grand on a boat rental, you can do what you want.

The crew guys came back and set up everything the same way. I kept my distance. Again! While I was swimming around in my ever shrinking beach area, a guy walked towards me that I haven't seen before. He was wearing one of the crew t-shirts and waved at me and yelled for me to come back on the beach.

I did and he said his name was Tom and shook my hand. He said I must have thought these people were a little rude yesterday for not offering me anything. I told him I didn't, they're doing their thing and I'm doing mine. He asked me if I wanted something cold to drink and of course, I said yes. My motto on these trips is I'll take anything that's offered, no matter what it is, even if I don't want it, I'LL TAKE IT!!

As we're walking towards where the big shots were, I asked him how he liked working for "that outfit" pointing at the yacht. He asked me "what do you mean?" I said to him that he looked like the cruise director or something like that and is it tough dealing with these rich guys that are quite demanding no doubt.

He looked at me and smiled and said "no, I don't work for them, I'm the rich guy who rented the yacht" and then he just laughed. I just looked at him and smiled and mustered up the most sheepish look possible. No matter, I met all his friends, got two packs of cigarettes and some French suntan lotion as well as some chilled bottled water and something to eat.

I also got a picture of me, Tom and two of his high-powered pals. When you look at the picture, you can obviously tell who the one guy is that doesn't fit in. Oh Britney, where were you when I needed you. Either way, they were all very nice and they left in the late afternoon. Ahhh, the beach is mine once again. Hope that's it for uninvited guests. Unless they come bearing gifts of course.

Day 9

Rained most of the day and a couple of boats anchored close by. There are two bikini "models" running up and down the beach. I tried not to stare too much.

Three goats were down sniffing around my tent. I chased them off. That must look so ridiculous if someone's watching. My fresh apples, bananas and 1 box of raison bran are finished as of today. Total supplies left? 11 cans of fruit cocktail, two boxes of raison bran and 35 liters of water that has to last 17 more days. Hmmm.

Day 10

"…Another fantasy bites…"

Both boats are gone. Had a huge storm last night that kept me up most of the night listening to the rain pounding on my tent. Shaved today. That was an experience. Bobbing up and down in three foot waves with a bar of soap in one hand and a Bic disposable in the other. No mirror of course. Didn't end up cutting my throat either. That's a good thing.

A tour boat called the "Wadadli Cats" pulled into my bay. As it was anchoring, it hit the bottom and made a hell of a screeching noise. All the tourists swam to shore, while the crew backed the boat off. Lots of bikinis running around. That always makes for a nice day.

One particularly attractive bikini walked right up and plunked herself down next to me. Oh boy, I thought, I wonder what she's offering. Don't see any cold water or cigarettes on her. She said Tom, the rich yacht guy told her about me and if the tour boat stopped here to say hi. Just hi? Another fantasy bites the dust.

Then some kid came over and asked me why I'm camped here. Then some guy comes over and asks how many days I have left here. Then one of the tour boat crew guys comes over and asks if I want anything. So much for nobody knowing I'm here! I very reluctantly declined his offer, they all said goodbye and they were gone. I'm exhausted now. Too much human interaction for one day.

Day 11

"...ricocheting bullets..."

I was sleeping and a woman's voice woke me up. A two mast schooner is anchored in my bay. Another bunch of boat renters. I did talk to them for a while, the Drake family from England. They offered me some food, but I passed that up for some cigarettes instead. The same still holds true that I think I mentioned somewhere before, I'd rather smoke than eat. A rather sorry state of affairs.

My bug bites are finally starting to heal, thanks to me using some insect repellent over the past few days.

And now, here's my worst nightmare come true. Heard a boat and voices around 4:30 pm. three guys in a boat heading over to the rocky area on the bluff beside me. One guy throws a plastic bottle on the rocks and then they backed the boat off around a 100 feet.

Out come the handguns with all three of them firing away. I was standing next to my tent so with the angle of the beach going slightly up and then dropping off to the water, they couldn't see me. They just continuously fired away and all I was thinking about was ricocheting bullets and my t-shirt drying in the tree next to me. If they had looked in my general direction they would certainly have seen that. The shooting stopped, boat revved and they were gone. Whew!

Day 12

"...it's New Year's Eve..."

Figure I'll try out that path I referred to earlier. There was an abandoned sugar mill about a half mile down and I kept going maybe another mile. That's enough, I'm worn out. Got back and my only souvenir was two giant blisters on both heels of my feet. Hiking and me? Don't agree. Of course, some sensible shoes might have helped.

When I got back, there was another boat anchored offshore. The owner was on the other end of the beach. I went swimming and saw him slowly walking back in my direction. He went behind me on the beach so I couldn't see him as I came out of the water. All I heard was a male voice say "hello." I turned around and met my first nudist.

How come there's no 20 year old female supermodel trying out the nudist look. I get a guy same age as me. He did give me the one thing that counted the most, a half pack of cigarettes. That was worth the encounter I guess, but a supermodel would have been much better I feel and I'm still wondering where he pulled that cigarette package from.

I must admit though, when there are no boats here, I've fallen into the habit of walking around and swimming with nothing on either. It is very liberating. It's raining hard again, and its New Year's Eve. I'll just sit here and stare at my two giant blisters.

Jan 1st 2006 day 13

"...the rum selection..."

Happy New Year! Well, another year has begun. All new trials and tribulations to face. Oh God! I've got 13 more days of this trial and trib and then back to the real world. That's even worse. Gave my head a quick shake as its only day one of a new year. My most pressing problem now? Getting all the damn sand out of my tent. If that my biggest problem of the New Year. I'd best SHUT UP!

A local showed up in the afternoon with his family. He owns a charter boat service and comes to this beach twice a month to get away from it all. Surprise, surprise. He looked at me in the beginning like I'd broken into his home and he'd caught me red-handed.

I left them alone like I do everyone else. When they were packing up go, he came over and asked me what I'm doing here. Gave him the standard explanation of getting away from it all and losing a few pounds to boot. I caved and asked him if he had any cigarettes, with no being the answer. But, he said the resort down past the nudist beach has a store and would I like a ride there. A STORE!! Don't have to ask me twice.

Next thing I know I'm in a sugar mill that had been converted into a store. Bought two packs of cigs, two diet cokes, one chocolate bar, one pack of Cracker Jacks and four tiny packs of cookies. (Are you starting to see the ongoing problem here?)

Also stared long and hard at the rum selection they had. I've been sober for almost five years now. If I caved just this one time way out here, who would know? Easy answer? I would! And I could never look someone in the face and say I've been sober since 2001. It's the only thing in my life, the ONLY thing, I've really truly stuck to and I'm not going to blow it now

Back in my tent, I thought I'd died and gone to heaven. Man that stuff was tasty! And I reflected on my decision with the rum. I was proud of myself today and I haven't felt that way in a long time. Not a bad start after all to a new year.

Day 14

"…poop on the beach…"

Rained hard all last night. At least this tent doesn't leak. Of course, I'd left my only two t-shirts outside to dry. Hahaha. Ended up sleeping in a black satin jacket I'd brought with me. How foolish must I have looked? It cleared up early and the suns out again. Got all my clothes dried out and the satin jacket is back in my pillow case. That pillow case was flat as a plate last night. Zero in it. My neck is killing me.

Around 11:00 am a bunch of crew guys from a sloop or schooner showed up. Woohoo! Britney finally showed up. Alas, was not to be, just another American businessman I'm told.

One of the crew guys, David, was from the Seychelles Islands. I'd thought about going there at one time, but camping is a big no-no. Anyway, as they were setting up, he gave some chilled water, apples, bananas and a beach ball. A beach ball? What am I supposed to do with that? Guess I could talk to it like Tom Hanks did in "Castaway." Nah, I'd never get that desperate. Would I?

The crew scurried about setting up tables and sun canopies for 11 guests. This time they did this right beside me, between me and the bluff. I asked one of the crew guys if the boat was owned or rented. Rented was the reply. I figured I had him beat with the 250 grand a week yacht that was here before. Wrong! This sucker costs $300,000 a week. I could live the rest of my life on that kind of money.

The guests were ferried in, all young, tanned and in fantastic shape. Men in Speedo's, women in bikinis. Wonder what I'd look like in a Speedo. Perish the thought!

There were a couple of kids as well. One of them immediately started running around on the beach. He looked down, then around and ran up to me. Wanted to know where all the poop on the beach came from. Don't look at me was my first thought. I told him there were horses running around here at night, must be from them.

Then this older guy was brought ashore. He must be the big cheese I'm thinking. He got out of the boat and with the kid still standing beside me shouts "Grandpa, this guy says there are horses running around on the beach." The old guy looks at the kid, then me and walks up to us. I'm sitting on the crest of this beach and he ends up standing beside me. I looked up at him, he looked down at me and said "wild horses around here?" I replied I didn't know if they were wild or not, but they keep me up at night sometimes. I pointed to the bluff to where the goats were grazing.

The older guy looks around and finally asks what I'm doing here. I gave him the standard reply and got the standard "this guy's nuts" look in return. He asked me where I'm from. Toronto Ontario is my usual answer, most people have heard of that. He said "oh, you must be a big hockey fan then, Eh?" I told him "no, I'm probably the only Canadian that isn't."

He looked down at me, stuck out his hand and said "that's too bad, my name is Ed Snyder, I own the Philadelphia Flyers." Even I'd heard of them. I replied "my name is Shannon, I'm unemployed."

"Unemployed?" He says, "how'd you get here then?" I couldn't resist. "Way cheaper than you did."

"...Arrivederci Bellissima..."

We both laughed, he took a look at my tent and asked what supplies I had. Time for some freebies I'm thinking. I told him I came here with just enough to last 25 days.

He thought about that for a second then told me a four or five star chef was coming onshore to make lunch for him and his pals. When they're done, I could help myself to the leftovers. Best invitation I've had yet.

I sat in my tent listening to the clinking of knives and forks on plates, just waiting for them to be done. Finally, they all got up and headed down the beach to walk off their lunch. Then, the most beautiful woman I'd seen in a long time appeared in front of me. One of the crew, she was Italian and apparently spoke no English. She motioned for me to come with her. I climbed out of my tent, she took me by the hand and walked me over to the table.

Mama Mia! Gourmet pizza, roasted ribs, baked potatoes, garlic bread and a bunch of other stuff I didn't recognize. Didn't care though. If it's good enough for Ed and his gang, it's good enough for me. I loaded it all up on an oversized monogrammed napkin and just as I was leaving, the Italian beauty dropped a grilled fish in with everything else. How'd I miss that? Back to my tent and chow down time. Man, it was good. Really, really good. Got enough here for tomorrow as well.

As Ed and his party walked down the beach, the crew started kicking my beach ball around. The Italian beauty has quite the kick to her. Then boom, my beach ball blew up and now I'll have no one to talk to tonight. Damn.

That was it, they packed up, I thanked Ed for his hospitality, waved goodbye to my Italian beauty and now it's just me and my broken ball. Arrivederci Bellissima.

Day 15

Guess what's for breakfast? Potatoes, garlic bread, rib and one grilled fish, after I flicked all the ants off first. Guess that's it for high quality eating for a while, unless Britney finally decides to make an appearance.

Two boats showed up while I was snoozing. Listening to them from my tent, they were obviously French. six men, six women (all topless, now we're talking) swam ashore and were having a little party. I made an appearance on the beach, they had a quick meeting, jumped in the water and swam back to their boats. That's gotta be a record for the French. Taking off when only up against one person, and I'm only HALF German.

Day 16

Two older folks from the nude beach swam around the bluff to my side today. At least they had swimsuits on. They said they just wanted to see what this side looked like. Uh-uh. And then they swam back. The excitement continues.

Went for a little snooze, but heard another boat pulling in my bay. Then silence. Then strange noises. I took a walk towards the beach, more strange noises getting louder now. Got to the crest of the beach just as it slopes down and what's going on? A couple of locals doing the "deed." Hmmm! I went back to my tent. I'd prefer to be in the show rather than watching it. OMG! He just made a mighty big noise. I think the shows over.

Day 17

Last night I think at least two horses had me surrounded, lots of snorting and crashing through the brush. Thought they were going to run right over me. It was a bit unnerving. I feel like I'm in Jurassic Park just waiting for some God-awful beast to stick its snout right through the tent flap. I took a couple of peeks out the flap, hoping to catch sight of one or more of these things.

At that moment, there was a bright light shining off the end of the bluff on my right. With imagination running wild, I figure there's two T-Rexes stomping around and a UFO off the end of the bluff. I laid back down, put a towel over my head and hoped for the best. And that was just last night. Today? Britney hasn't showed up yet and my tent's full of sand. Same old crap!

Day 18

"…how's it hanging?…"

Time for a foolish risk. The guy I hired to drop me off here and hopefully pick me up again was supposed to show up some time to check up on me. No show! I paid him the $75 for dropping me off, but kept the other $75 to make sure he comes back.

So I've decided to swim around the bluff to the nude beach and walk down to the resort where the sugar mill store is. I had two reasons for doing this. To see if there is an escape possibility if George doesn't show up and to resupply a little. Mainly cigarettes of course. Besides, if those two old gophers made it swimming around the point the other day, I should have no problem. Right?

Off I go in a t-shirt. shorts and my wallet in a Ziploc

bag. So here I am, swimming along if you can call it that, with one arm hoisted in the air holding a now leaking plastic bag and trying to swim with the other arm.

I reached the end of the bluff and crawled up on the rocks as I was beat. Next problem? Waves are coming in on a 45 degree angle and they are going to drive me right into the rocks. Not a good situation for a now, one-armed swimmer.

Off I go and end up banging and crashing into the rocks all the way from the point to the beach. My legs and one arm are all scraped up. My zip-loc bag is leaking badly. Oh no!! I'm rolling now with one wave after another driving me to shore, while trying to control myself with one arm.

I finally hit the shore, crawled up a few feet and flopped onto my back, my eyes closed. Well, now that was quite the experience, I'm thinking. Never done that before, and hopefully never again.

I open my eyes, look up and there's a naked man standing above me. His feet were on either side of my head and he's looking down at me. I blinked a few times taking in all the new sights and he says to me in a French accent, "where did you come from?" My response? "How's it hangin?" Still looking down at me, he replied "Pardon?" He used the French version of that word which to me sounded like "Pardo?"

He helped me to my feet and I explained I'd swam over from the other side of the bluff. He says "oh, you're the guy." Yup, I'm the guy all right, talking to a naked man with a leaky bag in my hand.

"...must have weighed 400 pounds..."

I sat on some rocks for a couple of minutes surmising my situation. My French friend left to continue his sunbathing and I am now faced with a decision I never in my life thought I'd ever have to make. I'm on a nude beach and now have to walk about a half mile to the resort. Do I keep my clothes on and look like a moron to all the people I pass by, or just grin and bare it, so to speak.

So with leaky bag in one hand and my shorts and t-shirt in the other, off I go. Oh My God! Not many people around at first, but as I got closer to the where the nude beach ends, there they were in all their glory. Average age of these people had to be a 100. What is it with the old people and nudity? They should be wearing six layers of clothes, not none. Looking around at the competition, I was feeling pretty good about myself. Passed one guy who had to be younger than me and he must have weighed 400 pounds. Yup, feeling pretty good. Maybe feeling adequate might be a better word. Not too fat, not too thin, not too tall, not too short and that one other thing that counts, at least where men are concerned.

Before you know it, the beach ends. Up a little path there's a sign that says, "Clothing must be worn beyond this point." With shirt and shorts back on, and I must say, back a little straighter, head a little higher, I walked through the resort and up to the sugar mill goodies store. I'm actually looking forward to my walk back now. Who would have thought!

My big question for these people here is, if George doesn't show on my scheduled extraction date, can I come here and get a ride or taxi back to St. John? The answer was a definite "yes!" Another problem solved, except to swim around that bluff again with all my gear will never happen. Most likely, I'd have to abandon most of it. I'll worry about that when the time comes.

I bought pretty much the same stuff I did last time I was here. Beverly, the lady running the store was eyeballing me all the time I was in there. I didn't exactly fit the look of an actual resort guest. I asked her to quadruple bag everything and explained how I'd gotten here. She looks at me, very disapprovingly I might add, and says "oh your that guy from over there," pointing in the direction of where I'd come from.

I just nodded and said "Ya, that's me" and started heading for the door. She grabbed me as I was leaving and pointed out a local who worked in the resort. His job, she told me, was to give lessons to the guests on how to use those surfboard things with the sail on them. She said the guy's name is Myron and maybe he'd give me a ride back. On a surfboard? How? I told her there's no way I'd get back on one of those things. She laughed and pointed out the full size motorboat anchored offshore. "No, in that" she says. I'm sold.

I went down there, explained to Myron what was going on and he said to give him a few minutes and he'd run me back. While I was waiting, one the resort guests came over to see who I was and I told him a couple of my stories over the past few days. He told me his name was Giles. I said "oh, the same name as the guy from Buffy the Vampire Slayer." He gave me a blank look, said "uhuh" and walked off. Not a big fan of the show, I'm assuming.

Myron's ready and 10 bucks later I'm back where I started. The best part of this is, he's going to pick me up on the 13th, bring me back to the resort and I can grab a taxi back to St. John. The 13th is a Friday. No pressure.

Day 19

Very sore from that swim yesterday. I don't think I'm going to do much of anything today. Oh. More noise on the beach, must be new tourists. They saw me and scattered. Time to read my Jackie Collins novel. Again! Same book I read when I first got here. I stupidly only brought four books.

Day 20

Everything becoming routine. Cleanup, exercise, and swim. I'm counting the days now. One week today I'll be home in my own bed. Gonna feel strange after sleeping on a bare tent floor with only a sleeping bag as a mattress.

I started eating the canned fruit cocktail today. I've only used four cans since I got here and it's all I've got left, food wise. Can't eat it though, way too syrupy. Cut one of the pockets out from inside the tent that has mesh on one side. Used it as a strainer and washed the fruit with some fresh water. Much more tasty now.

Day 21

"…My nudist days are over…"

Swam around the point again, both ways this time, just to see if I could. I wore a pair of running shoes because of the rocks and kept the cash in my pocket so I'd have two arms to swim with. I lost the shoes on the swim back. Walked the nude beach, feeling good again until I ran into three young local fellas. This time I was the, how shall I put this, the less desirable of the bunch walking around. I did the nude walk three times in total and that's it, no more. My nudist days are over.

I bought some goodies and quad-bagged them again for the trip back. Ran into Myron and sat with him for a while. He wanted to give me a ride back, but I told him I'd swim it. Also met some of the girls that work there, talked to them for a while as well. Most of the staff knows me now and I'm not even staying here. Well, I made it back. I am absolutely whacked. Bed early tonight.

Day 22

Major/major storm last night and I was awake through all of it. I am so tired and sore today, don't want to do much. Four days to go. Whooohoooo!

Day 23

Quiet day, just slept, swam or sat around.

Day 24

I'm bored stiff. No pesky tourists to deal with, no books to read twice! Just sat or swam. That's it. Watched the sun disappear into the ocean one last time and as I'm doing that, 30 feet away, six or seven pigs surrounded my tent looking for food I'm assuming. Good luck with that! It's my last night and I can't sleep. Tomorrow I'm free!

Day 25

Friday the 13th. Unlucky for some, not for me though. I hope. We'll see if Myron comes cruising around the point at noon. I'm packed up, cleaned up and I did my 25 days. First time I've set a time goal and actually did it. Feeling pretty good.

Myron showed up right on time, with company I might add. Two guests from the resort came over to see my side, a husband and wife from England. Introductions were made, I shook his hand and hugged his wife (a little too long from the look on his face) and told them the beach is theirs. Got into the boat, waved goodbye and off we go. Where's my hotel with the big comfy bed?

Aftermath

This is the first successful attempt at what I'm trying to do here. I lasted the full 25 days I'd planned and weighed in at 260 lbs when I got home. That's not bad I guess, but I always want more. Too much cheating while I was there would appear to be the problem. And I don't think I'll ever quit smoking.

I'm starting to think the only way this idea of mine would work and last a lifetime would be for me to build a one bedroom shack in one of these places I pick and stay there forever. I would end up being the skinniest, loneliest man on the planet. Hmmmm.

The drug guys came on a regular basis. They ignored me at first, but we were waving to each other by the time I left. I wonder what would have happened if they had come to pick up their stuff and one or all of their boxes were gone.

The names of the two yachts were the "High Chaparral" and the "Mirabella V" if you want to Google them and see what the big cash gets you.

Score: 1 ½ now out of 4 attempts. Yahoo!

Dominican Republic

"…and all would be well…"

Ahhh, the trip from hell. I was actually going to leave this entire section out because I didn't accomplish anything. To be quite honest here, I took next to no pictures, shot zero video and didn't even bother to keep a log. But I'm going to recap the entire experience for your enjoyment just so you can share my pain.

I flew out of Toronto in the early morning of Dec 31st 2007. I had not been feeling well prior to leaving for at least a month. I thought I had pneumonia or something like that. Went to the doctor a couple of times and was prescribed antibiotics which didn't seem to work. Don't forget dear reader, I still have the irregular heartbeat problem that medication has never quite controlled and also screwed up my first Costa Rican trip back in 2003.

And I still smoke as well. I know, I know. Say or think what you will. However, I did switch from regular cigarettes to lights. My doctor told me that would be ok. (I'm lying; she never said any such thing.)

So I land in the Dominican on New Year's Eve and hire a taxi to take me to a hotel I'd booked in advance. I was going to stay one night in the hotel, work my magic and find somebody to dump me off in the middle of nowhere. 26 days later this somebody would come back, pick me up and I'd be back in the hotel I started from. Airport the next day and home, maybe 20-30 lbs lighter and all would be well. Right? Wrong!

Jan 1st

"...appear to have grown clown feet..."

Woke up after a restless night and took a walk on the beach. Just up from where I was staying were a lot of boats that had been hauled up on the beach. I approached a couple of them and told them what I wanted to do, which in case you've forgotten is to find somewhere deserted and where I'd be left alone. One of them told me he knows of a spot and I hired him. We leave tomorrow. There is a grocery store just down the street from here so I'll hit that tomorrow first thing, stock up and off we go.

Also where I'm staying they have a café type deal out front so I thought I'd try that out. Sat down and ordered a tea and a bottle of water. A woman sitting at the next table over looks at me and asks "does that always happen to you when you fly?" Does what happen is all I'm thinking. So I have to ask "does what happen?" She replies "do your feet swell up like that after flying." Ok, what the hell is she talking about? So I look down and since last night or this morning, I appear to have grown clown feet. They are double the size of when I left.

I mumbled something to her, threw some cash on the table and went back into the hotel lobby. They have a gift shop in there with a full length mirror. Straight to it I go and I stand there looking at myself. Every part of me seems to have bloated up in the last 24 hours. I have no idea what's going on, but I still don't feel so hot.

I remember something about flying, prolonged sitting and water retention. No worries, among all the pills I take for my heart condition are water pills. Basically, I take these and can't leave the house for two hours. Very inconvenient. So I took a look through my medication stash, figured I'd pop a couple of those and problem solved. Wrong again. I forgot to pack them. Now I'm in real trouble.

So what's happening now is every drop of liquid that goes in, none comes out. No sweating, no washroom, no nothing. What to do, what to do? Go with the original plan I suppose.

Day 1

"…my heart was going to explode…"

Last night I couldn't sleep at all. I also couldn't lie down on the bed, I felt like I was drowning inside. Propped myself up against the headboard and spent the night sitting up. I'm starting to have trouble breathing as well. I figured the Dominican heat and air would clear up what was wrong with me. Only problem is its cool here and raining. Not helping my medical situation.

Big decision now. Do I carry on in this condition or scrub the entire trip? I'm supposed to meet the boat guys at noon and start this thing. I'm dumb, I'm here, let's do it!

Went to the grocery store, stocked up half-heartedly for 20+ days in the middle of nowhere, grabbed a cab and took the whole works over to the boat guys. I can tell I have a significant problem here because the head boat guy asked me if I was ok and if I really wanted to go through with this. My feeling still is if the weather clears and it gets nice and hot like it's supposed to be, this condition will clear itself up. So with that in mind, I told him lets go and off we went.

We went several kilometers down the coastline and he showed me several spots that looked like they would work. I was at the point of not actually caring anymore. I told him to pick somewhere and just drop me off. He did, right between two large resorts. I knew this locale would never work, too close to "civilization." I was so beyond the point of arguing over this. I told him this was fine, he and his pal dumped me off on the beach and left promising to return on the agreed pick-up date.

There was a small path running parallel to the beach behind me and a bunch of palm trees beyond that. I started to carry, then drag all my supplies and equipment over to the trees. I picked one and set up my tent behind it and covered the tent in dead palm leaves. Standing back on the path, I couldn't see my tent at all. All through this I thought my heart was going to explode right out of my chest.

In all honesty, I figured this was the end for me. I really thought I was gonna die here. I put all my supplies and gear in the tent and pretty much never left it again. I did the same I did in the hotel, propped myself in one corner with a bunch of stuff behind me. Anytime I did sleep, I did it sitting up.

Day 2

I am writing this from memory as I kept no written logs of anything. I don't really remember this day at all. I just remember eating nothing and drinking very little as I was having the same problem of everything in, nothing out. I didn't even smoke. I knew I was in very big trouble.

Day 3

"...two guns..."

This day I remember very clearly. Woke up still sitting up and it was raining. The weather hadn't gotten any better and I had gotten much worse. It was early in the morning and I pulled out my video camera to find out what day and time it was. I packed it back up and was just sitting in the tent staring into nothing and contemplating God knows what.

I heard something, so I looked out the tent flap at the ground. There out of nowhere were two pairs of shoes with feet in them and legs attached. I slowly lifted my gaze up the legs and stopped for a moment at the two guns in holsters strapped to two waists. I continued my upward gaze until I was looking at the faces of two policemen. Hmmm!

They started speaking to me in Spanish, which I still don't understand and most likely never will. I replied in English which I could see they didn't understand and so now we have a stalemate. They motioned for me to get out of the tent and of course, I didn't. Couldn't actually. They spoke, I spoke, lots of hand gesturing and unbelievably, they gave up and left. All I'm thinking is I should have gone with them, but I am too weak to do anything. This is gonna turn out so bad.

The rest of the day I did nothing. Just sat and thought of the opportunity I'd lost in the morning. I thought I was truly dead for sure as I am feeling worse and worse.

At 4:00 pm I heard a noise again and by my tent flap are those same two pairs of shoes. I look up at them, they look down at me. One of them pulls out a cell phone, dials a number, speaks for a few seconds and then hands the phone to me. It's their police chief who speaks English.

He wants to know what I'm doing here and specifically wants to know how I got here. I got the impression if I had have told him the truth of how I got here, he would have ordered his boys to go and find the boat guys and who knows what kind of trouble they would find themselves in.

"...robbers and murderers running around..."

So I played dumb (not so hard) and told him I hired a guy at random to drop me off here and that's that. I don't actually know anything else and most likely would never recognize him/them again. He accepted that sort of, but insisted I can no longer camp there as it's not allowed as well as being too dangerous. Too many robbers and murderers running around. Murderers? Really!!!

No matter, this is my free pass to get out of here and I took it. I explained to him my medical condition and he told me his men would take care of the situation. Good enough for me.

I passed the phone back and the policeman listened to his boss, nodding repeatedly. He hung up and both of them helped me out of the tent and as I sat on a rock, they proceeded to pack up all my stuff. As a gesture of thanks, I gave them pretty much everything, tent, food and water. I only kept personal items, much less for me to deal with. Everything went into their mini jeep (don't really know what the vehicle was) and off we went. One hour later, I'm back at the hotel I started at.

The owner of the hotel came out, took one look at me and helped me into her office. The room I had originally was gone, but she had a small one available if I wanted it. I took it. Straight to bed and OMG that was a long night.

Jan 5th 2008

Got up this morning after one of the worst nights of my life. I had little to no sleep whatsoever. As soon as I was able, I got on the phone to the airline I'd booked my flight with to change my return date. The person I got on the phone was extremely helpful and understanding and changed my return date to tomorrow.

Jan 6th 2008

Flight left the Dominican at 10:00 pm, arrived 1:00 am I think back in Toronto. The flight back was rough and it took me forever to walk through the airport. I was one of the last people to go through customs and surprisingly they didn't give me a hard time.

I remember walking back into my apartment at 3:30 am Monday Jan 7th. Home at last. Now I can die in my own bed. Well, that's how I felt.

Jan 7th 2008

Now I could have left the following out, but you really have to experience what an idiot I can be at times.

I'd taken some of those water pills I'd left behind, but they weren't working very well, so I got up at 9 am and called my doctor. I explained the situation to the receptionist and she booked me an appointment for 11 am today. I paused for a second and told her I was really tired from the flight and whatever and could she book me something for tomorrow instead. She rather reluctantly agreed and that was that. I'm booked in for 9:30 tomorrow morning. Figured I'd give those water pills of mine some extra time to kick in. mavbe I'd cure myself. I didn't!

Jan 8th 2008

Off to the doctor I go. I'm feeling no better at all and my pills are not working. I was led into my doctor's office and she was already sitting there. She took one look at me and said, "there's nothing I can for you."

That's reassuring I said or thought. She told me I had congestive heart failure (when the heart can't pump blood round fast enough to clear fluid from the tissues) and it's off to the hospital for me.

Aftermath

I went to the hospital that morning and 15 days later on Jan 22nd 2008, I walked out with a brand new pacemaker/defibrillator installed in my chest.

No more smoking I'm told. That lasted the 15 days I was in the hospital. I got out and went right back at it. Dumb/dumb/dumb! And I was told to watch my sodium intake, which is a crucial problem with the food choices out there. "Salt is my enemy." I'm still constantly telling myself that.

My weight ended up all over the place during this time, but I do remember getting weighed on my last day in the hospital and I was 268 lbs.

So, since I'd come back from the Costa Rican trip in 2003 I accomplished nothing. I'm back to square one. To quote myself from the beginning of this book "I came up with the idea in 1992 to stick myself somewhere isolated, make the source of my problems unavailable and I'd be cured." Obviously this idea does not work, and in Jan 2008 I gave up on this whole concept. I'm done.

Score: Still 1 ½ out of 5 attempts. No surprise.

Or am I?

Costa Rica 2010 Part 1

From Jan 2008 to June 2010 I scrapped my weight loss idea. I had totally given up and as many of you may be able to relate to, my weight over that time period slowly started creeping back up.

Strangely enough I knew it was, but didn't care anymore. I felt ok I kept telling myself. Pants got a little tighter. Shirt sizes starting going into the xxl and xxxl range. I still didn't care. Then something remarkable happened.

I had to get my driver's license and Ontario health card renewed in June 2009. I had to go to the offices of these places and have new ones set up as well as new photos taken.

When I received the new ones and looked at the pictures of me on them, I didn't know who this person was. Couldn't be me. I don't look like that. I compared them to my old licenses and the pictures did not look like the same person.

My face was so bloated out in the new pictures I just could not believe it. I stared at those pictures for almost 12 months and decided to resurrect my weight loss plan. I was in a different mindset this time. I truly had enough.

And with those pictures with me to look at every day, that's how I ended up back in Costa Rica in June of 2010 weighing in at a whopping 315 lbs determined to make this idea of mine work once and for all.

May 31st

Out of Toronto airport and onto El Salvador for a one hour pit stop and continued on to San Jose, Costa Rica, almost a carbon copy of the flight in 2003. On the flight from El Salvador the plane didn't have a lot of regular passengers aboard, but quite a few airline employees. Also, something that was most comforting, boarding out of El Salvador maybe 15 to 20 nuns and priests were on the flight. Don't know why, but I was feeling pretty safe about this flight.

Landed in San Jose around 4:00 pm local time and met up with John, a guy I'd found on the internet. His company is called "A Safe Passage." What he does is pick you up at the airport, take you to a hotel (it was nice), next day sets you up with whatever your travel plans are and sends you in the right direction. He does the same when you return. All airport transfers, two nights in a hotel and getting you setup to go to your next destination, $129 U.S. A fair deal I thought and it takes a lot of hassle out of the usual arrival and departure nonsense. Went to the hotel after stopping at a supermarket and crashed.

June 1st

"...$5 a night hotel..."

John picked me up in the morning and dropped me off at the appropriate bus stop which was on time and off I go to Liberia, Costa Rica. Five hours later I'm there. Grabbed a taxi and went the same hotel I'd stayed in on my 2003 trip. Didn't know what to expect, maybe it wasn't even there anymore. It was, with the same owner Dennis and the same wonderful ambiance you'd expect from a $5 a night hotel. The ambiance was the same, but the prices weren't. Up to $18 now, but there's a T.V in the room now and a frig and microwave in the lobby. For $13 bucks more, I'll take it, plus in all fairness the $5 rate was seven years ago.

I was much heavier than the last time he'd seen me so he was kind of surprised about that. You're not the only one buddy. I told him my plans on doing the same thing as I did in 2003, I just didn't want to go into Santa Rosa again, it's way too difficult getting in and out of there.

He recommended a place called Junquillal. It's another park, but there'd be no surfers there like last time and its rainy season again. So other than the park rangers on duty and the odd locals doing one day visits there, I should be pretty much alone. Sounds good to me I'm thinking, but I've heard all this before. We shall see. So I thought about it for about 10 seconds and agreed to give it a try, 28 days camped out in there.

He talked to one of his pals and he's going to drive me in for $38 U.S. That's a 50 kilometer trip one way. I told Dennis I'd have to stop at a supermarket first for supplies, how about $45 instead. A little extra for his pal waiting for me. Agreement all around, and my plan's in motion.

I took a quick walk over to the supermarket just to see what they've got and make a list out for tomorrow. Back to my $18 room with a color T.V.

Day 1

"…By sundown, I'm dead…"

I'm up early and ready to go. I think! Keep going over all the things that went wrong on the previous five attempts when I did this and I'm hoping I've got all the kinks worked out.

Ronny, my new and untested driver picked me up and off we went. First stop, a grocery store to stock up. Spent $84 on water and food basics. For 28 days, it doesn't seem like a lot. I'm also trying this with no cigarettes again. Probably a stupid thing to attempt yet again, but at least I have food this time!

Drove the 50 km to Junquillal. The road is not near as bad as the Santa Rosa trip in 2003. On the road in, we passed about a dozen vultures chowing down on a dead dog.

Got to the park and guess what? It's actually deserted. There's nobody here except me. Let's see how long that lasts. One of the park rangers, Randall, came over after Ronny left and helped me set the tent up. His English is pretty good, I do think he was told to look after me though.

There's a female park ranger here as well, older than me for sure. She was eyeballing me big time when I got here. I'll have to steer clear.

Swam all afternoon and by sundown, I'm dead. Unbelievably, even armed with a list, I forgot to bring or buy candles yet again. Sun goes down and that's it. No reading, no writing. Bed at 7:00 pm, up at 5:30 am. I'll have to figure a way to get my hands on some candles.

Day 2

"...She no understands..."

I was right about 5:30 am up. Rained on and off all day. Those vultures are trying to surround me, they only come near when I'm **in** the tent. Raccoons are sniffing around, iguanas out in force as well. I don't have any dry

134

clothes left. The rainy season is a little more intense than I remember in 2003. The Senora park ranger came over today with a cup of tea for me, then made her intentions quite clear.

No offence to anyone, but I'm not interested in a relationship with someone that appears to be older than my mother.(80) Only thing I could think of to tell her was that I'm gay. She no understands. God!! I pulled out my English/Spanish Dictionary which I made a point of bringing this time. Pointed to the word gay, which unfortunately, does not have the same definition as the one I was trying to put out there. Did some hand gesturing, she finally figured it out. Hope that puts an end to whatever she has in mind!

Day 3

Rain, rain go away. Come back in July. Nothing going on today. My lack of cigarettes is starting to take its toll however.

Day 4

It's actually nice for a brief time this morning with a gas powered weed eater as my alarm clock. A 6:00 am wakeup call I'd guess you'd call it. These park rangers are up and at em types. Two of them today, Senor and Senora park rangers. No relation, I just started referring to them that way for no reason whatsoever.

Guess I'll grab my wet swimsuit, wet towel and wet t-shirt and go for a swim. Started wearing a shirt as when the sun is actually out, I'm getting burnt big time. I'm using sun block 60, maybe need sun block 1 million. My nose as always is the first causality.

Day 5

There were some people here today. Locals with lots of kids. Parents look at me like I'm the grim reaper. Suppose I am from a looks standpoint. Remember, I was around 315 lbs when I got here. Not exactly a vision of loveliness. I brought five pineapples with me and have barely touched them. I don't like them really.

Day 6

Tent is a mess already; sand is my enemy once again. Grabbed one of those aforementioned pineapples, figured I'd give one a shot and ten thousand fruit flies came out of it. That's it! They must go. Gave one to the birds and the others to the park rangers. Senora park ranger thanked me profusely.

It's beautiful today, but starting to cloud over. It's only 9:30 am and I've been up since six. Oh, gonna be a long day. I can only amuse myself so much.

Day 7

"...naked Senora park ranger ..."

Think I got myself a ride to a supermarket four km away. I need those candles bad and time once again to cave in to the cigarette cravings. Like who am I kidding, I'll never quit. Only problem with the ride is it's one way, I'll have to walk back. Remember, I've been in the flooring installation business on and off for 41 years. My knees are not exactly in top notch shape, plus carrying all this excess weight around doesn't help either. I'll have to think about this. Four km! Yikes!!

Well, I took the ride, got what I needed and started walking back. Oh boy! Made it app two km I think and gave up. My legs are killing me. Found a path that led down to the beach and took it. From where I am now, I can see my tent. It's about the size of a postage stamp.

Walking is over for me, so I wrapped up everything in the grocery bags and tied them up. Shirt off, shoes and socks into shirt and tied that up as well. Into the water I go and I swam back. Visions of Antigua came racing back. Halfway back, my shirt seemed to get a little light. I turned around and one of my shoes was floating away and my socks were gone.

I hope there's no naked Frenchman waiting at the finish line. Maybe a naked Senora park ranger? I really hope not!

And I guess I'll have to fess up here. I bought a whack of cigarettes as well. The no smoking aspect of this trip is over!

Day 8

Clear skies today and man, am I burnt out from the walk/swim from yesterday. It rained real hard in the afternoon and evening, but at least I have candles now. Light at night. What a unique concept.

Day 9

One third of my time is done. Today I started my haphazard exercise program. I waited till today to lose some of the water weight everybody loses in the beginning of a diet plan. Now comes the grueling part, actual food reduction. I figure I'm going down to maybe 600 calories a day.

My exercise program mainly is a half-a** attempt at yoga, concentrating mostly on the legs. They are always sore. Usually after several days of constant swimming, I always feel better, I just don't carry it on when I get home. That's the one key thing I need to change in my life.

Day 10

Rainy season sucks. I've been stuck in my tent from 3:00 pm yesterday till today. It's like being in prison, only with an ocean 30 feet away. Ok, it's not like prison at all, but I bought the wrong sized tent. I usually get a 7 x 9 foot tent. This one is 6 x 8 and it's small inside. I'm living in an area of 48 sq/ft. No matter, I'll give this one away like I usually do and buy the right sized one for next time. If there is a next time.

Day 11

Another glorious weekend according to my little calendar. I have two more to cruise through. I can feel the changes weight-wise already and looking over the pictures I take on a daily basis, the changes are quite obvious. It will be very interesting to see what the final weight loss number is. This is my sixth attempt at this and I'm dead serious about it working this time.

I'm hoping to lose 30-40 on this trip. If I do I'm thinking about going home and coming right back down here for a second try. It would be so great to come in here at 315 lbs and go home in the 270 range.

Day 12

Should be family day here today, was four here yesterday, lots of screaming kids everywhere. Three cops showed up scanning the beach and water for…? I'm pretty sure I know what they're looking for, I'm just keeping to myself. Other than that, boring!

Day 13

Had to recharge my camera at the ranger station and while doing so, spotted four spider monkeys in the tree beside me. They looked down at me, I looked up at them. Very exciting. Yawn.

Hot and clear today for a change, I managed to wash all my clothes and dry them as well before the storm clouds rolled in and you know what started again.

Day 14

Ran out of bottled water today and I started drinking the water from the park taps. I'm told its ok, guess we shall see. I'm wondering what the sign beside the taps says though. It doesn't look like it reads "go ahead, drink this, you'll be fine."

Day 15

Well, today's the halfway point into my little jungle escapade. Waters drinkable I guess, I didn't sprout a third eye last night.

I'm down to a can of tuna or salmon in the morning and a protein powder drink in the afternoon. I also have four cans of fruit cocktail left and I think I'll save those as long as I can. My birthday is in 10 days and one can is reserved for that.

Police here again today with their machine guns, looking through their binoculars and scanning the bay. Must be a big shipment coming from Columbia going past here to all those nutcase Mexican gangs I've read about.

Day 17

"…a two foot water snake…"

Late last night woke up to hear a guitar playing. Where was that coming from? Was it real? I'd thought maybe I'd died in my sleep, but isn't it supposed to be a harp?

Nope, just some locals came in late, a momma, papa and one kid. When I came out of my tent, he came over and introduced himself. A fella named Luis and he wanted to know if I needed anything from the supermarket down the road. Do I!!

Hitched a ride and bought enough bottled water to last the rest of my time here. I'm sure the water here is fine, but I'm not taking any more chances.

Went swimming in the pm and as I was coming out of the water, beside me was a two foot water snake three feet from me. It was slithering along the sand in about three feet of water. As I made a 45 degree angle cut away walking out of the water, so did the snake staying with me. I waded onto shore and as a wave crashed on the beach, the head and half the snake's body poked out of the wave and I swear it was looking around.

Tell you where I went! Straight to my tent! I'm not going in that water again. THAT'S IT!!!

Day 18

"...an ant infested tent..."

I can't sleep worth a damn. Must be this no carb/high protein diet. Nights seem to last forever!

Went swimming this morning (that no more swimming thing didn't last long) and now I'm on the lookout for shark fins AND sea snakes. My head out there is bouncing around like a bobble doll steadily scanning for trouble.

And what's that? 10 feet away I see two little fins break water about four feet apart. Dumb as I am, I went for a closer look. Well, it's either a stingray or manta ray. Not sure, cause I didn't stick around long enough to find out. I'm not going in that water again. THAT'S IT!!! The only thing I haven't seen here is a shark, everything else is covered.

I talked to the park ranger when he moseyed by and asked him about the snake and sting/manta ray. He says they're harmless. I'm sure they are when you're standing on DRY LAND!!!

My digital camera I use for taking daily shots of myself is dead. DOA! Will not work. That's just great. I'll have to switch to my video camera, but I don't have anyone around to push the still photo button. I'll work it out.

Went back to an ant infested tent. Don't know why, don't know where they come from. Time to investigate.

Day 19

"...kept trying to taste me..."

Well, my digital camera is now officially dead. I started using the video camera today and with nobody to push the button, I just set it to record, walk in front of it and stand there like a fool. Hopefully I can retrieve still pix from the video. I honestly have no idea how this stuff works.

Couple of nice bikini babes showed later in the day. That was the thrill of the day.

Getting more tired as the days roll on, but my tans looking pretty decent though. At least that's something. Weight seems to be dropping off rather rapidly. Nothing wrong with that I'd say.

Senora park ranger back today, came over wanting to give me some Spanish lessons. I think she's still after something else, it's going to be a long afternoon.

Went swimming late pm and ended up surrounded by a school of tropical fish, like the type you'd see in a pet store. Little buggers kept trying to taste me.

Day 20

Had a large group of locals come in last night. Set up shop right beside me as usual. Even I recognized "happy birthday to you" sung in Spanish. Sounds much more sexy than the English version.

However, when the sun went down, they moved the party to their vehicles in the parking lot and as I'm writing this at 7:30 am today, the party is still happening. It was a very long night.

Back to my routine, maybe some sleep today hopefully. How come it didn't rain LAST night? Would have cleared them out fast enough I'm sure. Oh well, it's their country, not mine. Hola!

Now they're right beside me again. Spending the whole day here I suppose. I count 12 of them. Rain, please rain.

Slowly but surely they came over to introduce themselves and one very attractive chicka brought me a plate of food. Ok, now they're my friends.

And a few hours later they were gone, it's just me and the senora park ranger left. Ohoh!

Day 21

Nothing new, except for a massive storm last night. A huge tree beside the ranger station was hit by lightning and cracked in half. It took out a corner of the station. I woke to the sound of a chain saw. Normally, a woman on the end of a chainsaw would be kinda sexy. Not in this case. I really can't handle all this excitement. Haha!

Day 22

"...rather difficult to keep it up..."

Zero sleep last night and it's the first day of summer where I'm from. Not here though! It's my b/day in five days, that can of fruit cocktail is looking tasty. Went swimming with the senora park ranger in the rain. How romantic. When we were done, I walked back to the tent and she followed and crawled in right behind me.

I don't think she's buying the "I'm gay" story, but I'm sticking to it. She's caught me too many times checking out the bikini babes that wander around here at times. My head goes up like a giraffe when one is around.

After an awkward silence and firing up a cigarette in a very enclosed area, she left. Getting rather difficult to keep it up. The "I'm gay" storyline I mean. You knew that. Right?

Day 23

I'm in a groove now. Swimming and my version of yoga, reading, writing and more swimming.

Lay awake most of last night working on another idea for a book tentatively called "The Genesis Concept." Nothing more to say on that subject. It's amazing how many ideas can flow through your head in a place like this. Mostly bad!!

Day 24

Wondering about getting picked up on June 30th. With all this rain, the road is very bad. Every time I've done this, getting out looks to be a problem as the days count down and I can never get it out of my head.

Five cops in a boat just showed up. They anchored it, went overboard and with revolvers and machine guns in the air, waded onto shore. Felt like a mini invasion. It's only me here, heavily armed as well with a can opener and a plastic spoon.

Three of them went to the ranger station; the other two stayed and guarded the shoreline. I feel so safe. Five cops, three park rangers and me. The cops took off and the rangers showed up with tea and biscuit's. Biscuits?

Senora park ranger showed up at my tent last night in the rain. She's just not gonna give up and I'm not gonna give in. I'm not that easy. Hahahahaha.

Day 25

"...how's Lindsay Lohan doing..."

Starting to get to the point it rains every day with thunder and lightning. One of the rangers told me today the road is worse than ever. One of them was scheduled for pickup yesterday and the truck couldn't get in. Four kilometers out of here. With everything I'd have to carry, I'd never make it. How many times have I faced this decision only to have everything work out. Hope for the best I guess.

Ran out of water again today. Guess I miscalculated that big time yet again. Back to park water. Ugh!!

Late in the day a group showed up, three guys, three girls. How did they manage the road in, I thought it was horrifying. They jumped around in the water and all spoke English. A refreshing change. When the oldest guy of the group walked past me, he gave me a nod and I asked him how bad the road is and if anything interesting was happening in the world. He came and sat down with me and told me he doesn't watch the news, too depressing. I can relate to that. The road isn't so terrible, he added. That's good news I guess.

He asked what I was doing here and I gave him the condensed version. He gave the same look most people do and asked where I was from. Hamilton, Ontario, Canada I replied and turns out he's from Windsor, Ontario, not all that far from me.

I can't remember the following exactly as I kinda zoned out as he was speaking, but I think he's a PHD or professor of some kind somewhere and he's been here three months and is going home soon. On and on he went.

When that was done he asked about my food supply and I gave the standard response that "I'd rather smoke than eat" and ran out of cigs a long time ago. He amazingly offered to come back tomorrow (maybe) and bring me some goodies (his words) and some cigarettes. An offer I can't refuse.

I know I'll never see this guy again, but I put in an order for four packs of cigs and whatever food. I explained about my half-baked attempt at a high protein, low carb diet and I thought that was it. He started on about something else and went on and on. I'd finally had enough and it was getting dark so I asked the big question, the one I knew would get him moving. "By the way, how's Lindsay Lohan doing, last I heard she got some problems."

He looked at me blankly, said "who?" and decided he'd better get going. Bye, bye. See you tomorrow. Not likely!

Day 26

"…it's Mr. Windsor…"

The day before my birthday. No bottled water, one can of fruit cocktail earmarked for tomorrow, half dozen cans of tuna and salmon, protein drink mixed with park water. Things are peachy. Ugh!!!!

Other than my routine, I didn't do anything except keep looking up towards the road occasionally. Guess Mr. Windsor aint coming. Oh well, five more days and I'm outta here.

Went for a sunset swim and after sitting next to my tent, I heard a vehicle coming. Can it be? Sure enough it's Mr. Windsor. I can't believe it. He jumped out of the truck and walked towards me with a bag swinging in his hand.

Oh, it's like Christmas.

He came over and sat across from me and handed me the bag. I could have kissed him. If I was really going to, I would have made sure Senora park ranger was watching. Put that situation to bed, so to speak.

I opened the bag and rooted through it and guess what? No cigarettes. Some meat, cheese, fruit and bread. Well, he got the food part half right. So I asked him where the cigarettes are. He told me HE decided I was better without them and didn't buy any. HE decided. Hmmm. How does one respond to that? One doesn't. I asked him how much I owed him, paid him, thanked him and off he went.

So Mr. Windsor. Mr. I Know Best. Mr. Holier Than Thou. I have not used any offensive language throughout this entire book and will not start now. You can pick whatever nasty words you can think of and insert them anywhere you like.

Mr. Windsor, you are without a doubt the most presumptuous, arrogant, pompous, piece of work I've ever met. I could tell just from our first few minutes spent together talking you think your better than everybody else, better educated and better whatever.

You were the oldest of the group you were with and I can only hope none of the three young girls are involved with you. @!#$ &*#. See if your mammoth brain can decipher that.

Day 27

I'm getting out of here. That douchebag from yesterday has done me in. I gave the fruit and bread to the rangers and asked them to fire up the cellphones and get me out of here. No cigs. next to no food. Had enough. It's my birthday today. Whoohoo. My b/day gift to myself? Get the hell outta here.

Ok, I'm calmer now. Time to re-evaluate. Ok, one of the park rangers friends showed up on a dirt bike. They both came down to see me and $10 and an hour later, I've got five packs of cigarettes. Best b/day gift I ever got. Turned out to be a lovely day after all. Screw you Mr. Windsor.

Day 28

Rained hard last night and into the morning then it cleared up. And thank God for that, as almost everything I own is soaked. Clothes, bedding, everything. The tent leaks where the floor is sewn to the walls, a distance of five inches. It rains so hard the water gets kicked up that high.

Met a family here for the day from San Jose. We chatted for one hour and the two bikini clad daughters were gorgeous. I'm sure the Senora park ranger is eying this situation from afar.

One of then spoke passable English, the other not so much. I finally got around to asking how old they are. 14 and 15 was the reply. YIKES! The mom was pretty cute as well. How do I get rid of him I'm thinking. And then they said goodbye and left. Hmmmm.

Day 29

One of the rangers woke me up late last night to walk down the beach where a sea turtle had come ashore to lay eggs. I grabbed my video camera, but I knew it was way too dark.

He shone his flashlight on the turtle, which didn't like that at all while I tried my camera. No go. The turtle was enormous and I had never seen one of these close up before. Pretty impressive. Not sure why it's here now though. I don't think it's the right time for sea turtles. Ah, what do I know.

All I did today was work on my "I wanna be on Survivor" video. This is gonna suck big time.

The other thing I did was worry about being picked up in two days. I seriously have got to stop cutting this so close. We shall see.

Day 30

This is my last full day here. Scheduled pickup is tomorrow at noon. I'm going to get the ranger to use his cell phone and confirm this, but if my ride is available, I'll get him to come today.

My ride is not available, but the ranger called his friend Antonio and he's going to get me out of here today and give me a ride to Liberia. Whoohoo! Freedom. Tony showed up as promised and at 2:00pm, I'm back in Liberia.

One thing I know for sure is I lost weight big time this time around. I guess that's it for this camping experience.

Aftermath

Got home and total weight loss was 40 lbs exactly. Finally, a real success. Now I get to do this all over again in 2 months.

When I left for the second part of this, I'd actually managed to keep the 40 lbs off. Things are looking good.

Score: 2 ½ out of 6 attempts. Yaaay!

Costa Rica Part 2

Sept 2nd/3rd

I arrived in San Jose and went through the same routine as two months ago. Stayed in the same place and took the same bus to Liberia after grabbing one of the last two seats. After that it was standing room only. Imagine standing in a bus for 228 kilometers. Back the same hotel there and booked the same driver I had last time for tomorrow. This is starting to get boring. And I need to find a replacement for the word "same."

Day 1

"...hug and kiss..."

Packed up this morning, hit the grocery store (same one if you hadn't guessed already) and off to the park. Started down the four kilometer dirt road and partway in we passed two policemen standing on the side of the road looking out into a field. We both thought they were on official business, and other than Ronny saying hello, we continued on.

We got to the park and my female park ranger pal was on duty. Got a massive hug and kiss from her while her colleague stood there smirking at me. I'll have to evade her somehow for the next few days. I got the same campsite spot as the park was totally deserted again. Not bad. So far.

The two policemen walked up to where I and the two park rangers were sitting and plunked themselves down. One of them I recognized.

Found out they had walked the four km mud-pit road into the park. I asked them why and was told their truck was broken down and the department didn't have the money to fix it. Now that's a budgetary problem for sure!

Actually I thought they were both kidding, but I looked around for their truck and it wasn't there. Kinda felt sorry for them. The five of us set up my tent and put everything away and then they disappeared. Once again I'm alone.

Day 2

Big, big storm last night, the tent was bent over sideways. Thought I was going to lose it. Made it through though, got a little water leakage around the zippers. All I'm thinking is nothing has changed; it's like I never left for two months. Nothing much happening today, just getting back into the swing of things here.

Day 3

Senora park ranger brought me lunch today, grilled fish and salad. So much for evasion tactics. By the time I get out of here, I'll be married.

Started my usual exercise program again. My version of yoga for the legs and sit-ups. Gotta keep trying to flatten the gut out. With 40 lbs off the first trip, have to try and do it again. I don't see another 40 off though, but anything's an improvement. I've got 32 days left to see some real results. Not eating much really, something about the atmosphere here, don't think about food much. That's a good thing I suppose.

Cleaned out the tent today with my mini whisk broom and dustpan. Best piece of equipment I ever bought. Only took seven times doing this to work the kinks out and bring stuff I actually need.

Day 4

Today I broke the clippers out I'd purposely brought with me and shaved my head, but not before giving myself a Mohawk first. A 56 year old stuck here and when will I ever have the opportunity to do this again? Never!

I videotaped the whole thing and will post it somewhere someday. It was quite frightful looking. Not a good look for me. I also taped whales offshore. They were very close. Hope it turns out.

Truckload of people showed up, similar group from the last time I was here and they pretty much ignored me just as much as last time. I don't think I even mention them in Part 1. That's how much of an impact we had on each other.

My senora park ranger stalker is gone, she's off duty for a few days. I'm safe for a while. No sooner did I think that and the guy ranger shows up with a cup of tea for me. How delightful! He's gone in five days.

Day 5

Didn't do much of anything today. Worked on this and tried to get my netbook charged up but it's so cloudy here the ranger stations solar batteries were low so no charging available today. Great!

Day 6

Whales have invaded the bay here. They are everywhere. Got lots of video of them. Fins and tails out of the water, some as close as 300 feet offshore.

I'm surrounded once again. two guys came in on a boat late last night and set up right next to me. Then early this morning 10 students hiked in and set up on the other side of me. Nice big deserted park here and it's "one, two, three in a row!" I don't get it. Spread out a little. Besides, they're noisy as hell.

Day 7

Boat guys next to me were yapping all night last night. No sleep for me. Students running amok all day. No sleep for me. Went to the ranger station to check out the solar situation. No recharging for me. The day's a bust. Into the tent, pillow over my head and that's that!

Day 8

Things are looking up. Woke up this morning and the students and boat guys are gone. Got the place to myself again. 10 minutes later a bunch of locals showed up, their trucks and themselves all covered in mud. That's a shame. The road in must be getting worse. I think I'll go investigate.

Took a walk up to the station with netbook in hand hoping to recharge this thing. Whoohoo! Their solar batteries are charged and so will my comp in a couple of hours.

Plugged it in and took a walk up to the park entrance to check the road out. The two male park rangers went with me. There's two here now on full time duty.

At the entrance is a little bridge and the road leading up to it is now a deep mud pit. I suggested to the boys that if they have nothing to do why not fill them in. They both laughed and we went for a cup of tea. Netbook is recharged, I actually accomplished something today.

Day 9

The mud covered locals stayed here last night. Looks like they slept in their vehicles. Guess they were afraid to chance the road again after yesterday. Boohoo! One of the vehicles car alarms kept going off last night. Sounds like being back home, except for the constant bug noises and waves crashing on the beach.

Day 10

Comp is dead again and no sun out today. That'll be bad. There's a 10 ½ hour battery in this thing, but it sure don't last that long. Well, I'll check out the station and see what's up. It was easier when I just kept notes and redid them at home, as long as I don't lose them of course!

Senora park ranger is back on duty today and she doesn't like my new hairdo. We're not ever married yet and I'm getting those looks I remember so well. The bloom might be off the rose, so to speak.

Day 11

"...Never talked. Never touched..."

I was wrong about de-blooming the rose. Last night after the sun was down and pitch black out, she showed up at my tent, opened it up and made herself at home. I was reading by candlelight and she brought a pillow and blanket, spread it out and laid down. Hmmm.

Now the next part I'm sure will insult someone reading this, but quite frankly, I don't care. I said to friends and family on several occasions maybe one day I'll come back from one of these trips with a 20 year old wife that speaks no English. That way I don't have to listen to anything. It was never my intention to come back with one older than me. Bigger too!

So that was about the most awkward night I ever spent in my live. Never talked. Never touched. She must have really wondered what's wrong with Canadian men. Nothing, they just don't want to be involved with someone that looks older than their mothers. Enough said on this, I just wonder how the rest of my time is going to go here. I have 19 days left to go. GOD!!

Day 12

Got up this morning and nobody's around, if you know who I mean. I just carried on with my regular morning routine. Cleaned the tent out and laid low for the entire day. She never showed up. On well, no more tea and fish for me I suppose.

Day 13

Senora park ranger showed up this morning with a cup of tea and not a word was spoken of the non-event from two nights ago. We just kinda sat staring into nowhere, an uncomfortable situation to say the least.

She finally left and I started doing my usual daily ritual. Cleaning, writing, sleeping swimming. Day done.

Day 14

"...She's dickin with me..."

Two weeks down, how many to go? And here's a fascinating turn of events. I'm told now that the park is closed because the water is "sick." What does that mean? I know there's been a lot of dead fish washing up on shore, but why now? I have to leave? I've been dumped by a relationship gone bad before, but thrown out of a national park? A new low for me.

I've seen them collecting water samples on a regular basis and some park people have come to pick them up. Some of the samples I've gotten for them. Hah! Send in the Canadian to do the dirty work. Senora park ranger says the water smells bad. I don't smell anything. She's dickin with me I think since I wouldn't return the favor. Oh God!

So now I got Senora park ranger playing mind games with me and now the other male ranger shows up and tells me "no swimming." They're in cahoots these two. I'm not sure if he's serious or not, cause he's always smiling. I felt ok, so I'm not sure what to do. I know. I'll ignore the pair of them.

They were told by park officials I found out, that its ok for me to stay, but nobody else is allowed it. I'll take that. Swim, swim all day long. I have gold plated travel insurance, course by the time whatever God-awful symptoms show up, I'll be as goner. Closest hospital is 50 km away and there's no way out of here.

Hear that Mark Burnet, head Survivor honcho? No helicopter behind the hill, no medics hiding behind the trees. Anything happens here, odious amigo.

156

Day 15

Well, so much for the park being closed. I get up this morning and there's a family camped next to me. Dad, mom and two little kids. Closed. Right!

None of them are swimming though, just me. Medic! You gotta take your chances. Still don't know what the water problem is, nobody here to explain anything. Fish are still washing up on the beach and even the vultures aren't touching them. That's a very bad sign. I'll just carry on as usual, as long as blood doesn't start washing up on the beach, I'm not worried.

Day 16

"...was kinda cute..."

Senora park ranger brought me a lunch today. I guess all is forgiven. Unless she poisoned it! Grilled fish (maybe one of the dead ones) and hot peppers. Wherever it came from, it was delicious. I don't feel so good. Just kidding.

Ridiculous story of the day? I went for a snooze in the afternoon. The family beside me is gone and now I'm all alone again. So as is usually the case, I got up and climbed out of the tent wearing just my underwear.

The tent front is facing the ocean, so I climbed out, zipped the tent closed and walked around the side of the tent and literally bumped into four nuns wearing the full nunnery gear. I stood there in my underwear, they stood six feet in front of me and all I could think to say was "hi." They stood there frozen on the spot and my next word? "Bye."

I turned and back into the tent I go. My only thought as I sat down in the tent was and I swear to God this is true (I will be damned for all time now) was "the one on the left was kinda cute." Yes, damned indeed. Maybe I've been here too long.

Day 17

Spent most of the day writing about my previous trip here into my comp, which is once again fully charged. Also, listened to a gas powered weed eater all day long. Guess it's park lawn maintenance time. Two bikinis showed up in the afternoon, something nice to look at for a while.

Day 18

Senor park ranger fired up the weed eater again at 7am. Makes for an interesting alarm clock. In any of my previous trips and logs, you've listened to me whining constantly about rain, rain, rain. Well, don't know what happening here, but it's been rain free for three days. A most welcome change. I'm told the dry season starts in Dec and ends in April, so at this point I'll take anything. Guess I'll go recharge the netbook, nothing else to do.

Day 19

"...best of friends, right?..."

Senior park representatives showed up today to check the area out and talk to the people here about their impressions of the place. Since I'm the only people here, I guess I'm it.

The rep that came over to talk to me was an absolute cutie, spoke English and was quite happy I gave the place high marks. Senora park ranger kept quite close to monitor the situation. The rep said she remembered me from June and was quite pleased I'd come back again. Hold on! I don't remember her at all. What's up with that!

We talked for a while about life in Costa Rica and Canada. I got out of her she was single and unattached, but really, what good does that do me here? None! Keep dreaming I tell myself. Only one real point I wanted to make though.

Senora park ranger was a dozen feet away standing there listening to a conversation totally in English. I knew she could pick up bits and pieces, but not much else. So I walked over to her, put my arm around her and told "cutie" that Senora was the reason that this park runs so well and without her it would all fall apart. Everybody's all smiles now and I said aloud with my arm still around her that we are "best of friends, right?" and repeated the word "RIGHT?" Senora said "Si, yes" and hopefully that ends that!!! (It did)

Day 20

Started working on my Survivor audition video speech today. I'm planning on taping that on my last day. That will also be the day I get to finally shave all this crap off my face. I hate beards, especially on me.

Had the landscaper in today. Did a beautiful job. My little area is about 30 x 50 feet and he just blew through here with his weed eater. Looks absolutely fabulous!

Day 21

Three weeks down and two to go. The rain is back with a vengeance. So much for early dry season theory.

Rained all night and still is as of 11 am.

Later in the day I taped what I think are porpoises swimming close to shore, maybe a 100 feet away. There are three buoys off shore, about 150 feet away when the tide is out and every day I would swim out to them, touch one and swim back. When I saw those fins poking out of the water between the beach and the buoys, that ended that exercise program.

Went out around 4 pm for my final swim of the day, not too far this time and ended up laying on my back with my ears underwater, I could hear the whales that are constantly offshore talking to each other. Whale music I believe it's called. Very soothing.

Day 22

Rained all night and into today again. Gonna be a long day, comp needs recharging and all three of the books I brought with me have been read. Oh boy! Time to lie down and stare at the top of the tent.

Day 23

I won't even bring up the rain factor again. I'm wondering if a tropical storm or a hurricane blew through the Atlantic side and we're getting some pieces of it. In all the times I've been here, I've never seen it this bad. Something's up.

I hear a voice. It's in my head. "Some chocolate covered almonds would be nice right about now." SHUT UP!!!!!

Day 24

Cleared up enough this morning that I could dry out everything I own. The moisture in the air is leaving everything damp. Clothes, bedding, my one and only towel. Everything.

Around noon the storm clouds moved in again. I grabbed all my still wet stuff out of the trees and headed for the tent. Time to hunker down for the day.

Day 25

Don't know why but I was really sick last night. Some stomach thing. My food supplies are down to the cans of tuna and salmon, maybe one was off. Gonna lay down the rest of the day. UGGGG!!

Day 26

Still feeling the effects of yesterday. I'm thinking now maybe I'll skip the eating for the next few days. I did it for 15 or 16 days on my first trip here in 2003. A few more won't kill me. I think.

I'll see if I can survive on water, gum and toothpicks. Hmmm. Do this till Oct 8th? Marvelous. Should be good for a quick 10 lbs extra off. We shall see.

Day 27

"...With arms flailing..."

Yesterday was day one completed of my three day gum and toothpick diet plan. Feeling ok. Swimming has been curtailed here. The surf is just pounding the beach.

Going in, it's difficult just getting past the waves. I was hit with one and it just picked me up and slammed me back onto the beach. That's enough of that nonsense!

Weathers still lousy and it's raining on and off, but the winds coming off the ocean are getting stronger. I was in the tent in the morning, sitting there watching the waves through the tent flap when the wind caught the screened in area on the front of the tent. The wind yanked the tent pegs out of the ground and blew the entire front of the tent right at me while I sitting inside the sleeping area. It bent the top of the tent right down so I ended up laying on the floor with the top of the tent a foot from my face. Very exciting!

Winds died down for now. I hope! Climbed out and surveyed the damage. Tent's in one piece, so I put it back up again. The screened in area on the front of the tent has mesh you can look out of, with blinds on each screen that can be rolled up or down for privacy. I rolled them up on Sept 4th when I got here and never touched them again.

Thought I'd roll them down to dry them out. Rolled down the big one in the very front and a million red army ants went nuts. Yikes!! Seems I disturbed their new home. These things took off in all directions at the same time a gust of wind grabbed the flap they were on and flapped it up and down a few times. Next thing I know I'm totally covered in these things and, man, do they bite!

With arms flailing, trying to get these things off me, I ran into the ocean, screaming like a little girl. Ahhh, the joys of camping. And thank God there was nobody around with a video camera to witness that. Not exactly what I'd want to see posted on YouTube. It must have looked pretty funny though. I'm tired!

Day 28

Winds and rain are bad again. The front of the tent blew out of the ground again last night. Kind of annoying. Put it all back together in the dark.

Two guys walked in and came down to the beach covered in mud. They walked straight into the ocean, clothes and all. Senora park ranger came down to check them out all dressed in her finest rain gear.

They all came over to my tent and we sat in the screened in part. It didn't do much good cause the rain was coming down sideways. I'd put some heavy logs and stones on top of the tent pegs hoping that would hold everything in place. It did.

Seems they'd tried their luck with the road in a regular car (not a good idea), and it was stuck in a mud-pit. Alarm bells start going off in my head. All I ever think about towards the end of one of these little excursions is if I'll be able to get out of here on time. Always worries the hell out of me. I always time everything too close together. Pick-up, traveling time and hit the airport sometimes in the space of 24 hours. I know it's not a bright idea to plan everything so tight and still, I do it every time

They all went back to the ranger station and I sat there deciding my next move. Didn't take too long to decide. Time to get out of here, before it ends up not being a possibility. I'll start extraction plans tomorrow.

Day 29

I'm flying out of San Jose on Oct 10th, so I have six days max to get out of here. I was originally going to stay in this park for 35 days. If I have to cut it a little short, so be it.

Those guys must have got their car out either last night or sometime today, cause I never saw them again. And now I have to talk to Senor park ranger about using his cell phone to call the guys that got me in here. I did. He tried. Don't work. No reception. So, through the park radio system, they got hold of Dennis and he's going to come in late tomorrow. He has a four-wheeler and hopefully he'll make it through. We'll see tomorrow.

Day 30

Tent's still standing. All my stuff is soaked. I've kinda taken up residence in the middle of the tent as that's the only dry spot left. And what happens around noon? It clears up completely. Ya, the calm before the next storm I'll bet. Took all my stuff and hung it outside everywhere. Two hours later and it's all dry. When the sun is out, it's blazing.

I packed everything up, except the tent which I've given to Senora park ranger as a consolation gift and who is off duty. She comes back tomorrow, so I don't have to face that if I get out of here today. So with the tent still standing, I took all my stuff up the ranger station. No sooner had I got there, Dennis drove up, his truck covered in mud. Hope the cleaning bill is included in the transport costs.

I thanked both the guy park rangers on duty, told them to give Senora park ranger my regrets for missing her, climbed into Dennis's truck and off we go.

The road had dried slightly but was still a major mess. In spots, some of the road was gone. It had just broken off and fallen down the drop off beside us. Four km later and we're back on solid ground. That's it!

Oct 4th-10th

After recovering from my 30 days in Junquillal, I hired Ronny, the guy that took me into Junquillal on day one, and we went waterfall hunting over a few days. Found some beautiful ones and one, which I can't remember the name of, we spent a half day at. Ronny was bored, but I enjoyed it.

On the 9th, I took the bus back to San Jose, stayed in the same hotel John had arranged for me and on the 10th, airport and home.

Aftermath

Weighed myself when I got home and I'd dropped another 20 lbs. Not bad, 60 lbs over the course of the summer. No success as far as quitting smoking goes though. One thing at a time I suppose.

So I weighed in at 315 when I left on May 31st 2010 and was down to 255 on Oct 10th. 60 lbs off in total and I'll take it. Trick is now to keep it off. I went against my own advice from my introduction and joined the local YMCA. I'm not much for the exercising stuff, but I am in the pool every day. Gotta start somewhere, right?

And I know the smoking has to come to an end. My biggest fear is quitting and ending weighing 500 lbs. OMG! What a horrible thought. Think how many trips I'd have to take to lose that kind of poundage. Hmmm. That's it.

Score: 3 ½ now out of 7 attempts.
(I'm on a roll.)

Krakatau Volcano, Indonesia

Sundra Strait, West Java

This is a place I've wanted to visit for a very, very long time. The Krakatoa volcano has fascinated me only because of the destructive power that it unleashed so long ago. By long ago, I mean 128 years ago. In 1883 it erupted and literary blew itself to bits. The damage it caused was catastrophic. The following is a short history of Krakatoa that I found on the internet.

"…killed more than 36,000 people…"

There were four gigantic explosions on August 26 and 27 in 1883. A black cloud of ash rose 17 miles above Krakatoa and that cloud from the eruption of Krakatoa spewed around 11 cubic miles of ash into the atmosphere.

On August 27, more violent eruptions occurred, and one of them blew away two-thirds of the island. This was one of the most deadly volcanic explosions on Earth in recent history. It was this explosion and collapse of Krakatoa that generated tsunami waves as high as 120 ft.

These waves killed more than 36,000 people along the coastlines of Java and Sumatra. The tsunami waves also were seen in the Indian Ocean, the Pacific Ocean and along the North and South American coastlines.

The 1883 eruption of Krakatoa was given a Volcanic Explosivity Index of 6 which rates it as "colossal." The 1883 eruption was equivalent to 200 megatons of TNT. In comparison, the Hiroshima atomic bomb was only about 20 kilotons.

In 1927, underwater eruptions marked the unexpected appearance of Anak Krakatau (Child of Krakatoa) which

166

has since risen out of the sea, reaching a height of around 800-1000 feet today. Here are a couple of recent activity reports of Anak Krakatau I found in the Jakarta Post newspaper.

"Mount Anak Krakatau continued on Sunday its frenzied expulsion of volcanic material, including hot rocks, sand and dust shrouded in toxic fumes — seven times more frequently than just a week earlier."

"Usually Mt. Anak Krakatau experiences an average of 90 to 100 small scale eruptions a day. Now, the number of eruptions can reach 700 a day,"

"...let's go camp out on this thing..."

Why wouldn't any rational, sane person not want to see this monster up close? All I can think of is, "let's go camp out on this thing. What could possibly go wrong?" My ultimate goal is to camp out on the one remaining piece of the original volcano. I figure two weeks camping is enough and on this trip I don't care if I lose a single ounce, I've just got to do this. So in Feb 2011, I booked a flight and on March 7th I left. Return date is March 22nd.

I booked all car transfers and hotel accommodations in advance, something I don't normally do.

"...It's a smokers paradise..."

I left my home at 3:15 am on March 7th and walked into the hotel in Jakarta Indonesia on March 9th at 12:17am. Total traveling time was 33 hours after factoring the time zones and dateline crossing. I think that's right.

My first observation after settling in here? It's a

smokers paradise. Take all the anti-smoking laws in place in Canada, particularly Ontario where I hail from, take all the laws, which I believe border on a police state mentality in some cases, take all of them and reverse them 180 degrees. If you don't smoke here there is really something wrong with you. At least here, I'm not treated as the anti-Christ because I choose to use a legal product. Well, enough on that.

I was tired but not wiped out by the jet lag. I spent one night in the hotel in Jakarta and left for Carita Beach just after 11:00 am and it's still March 9th.

The driver that was hired amazingly was the spitting image of Hosni Mubarak, former President of Egypt. So this is where he disappeared to? Used to rule an entire country and now he's driving me around Indonesia? I called him El Presidente from this day forward. Don't know why, that's the Spanish version, but he thought it was funny.

I came here only with U.S $ which surprisingly, they don't seem to want. I exchanged $500 U.S into local currency and another of my life dreams came true, because no matter how fake or fleeting, for a while I was a multimillionaire.

$500 U.S exchanged for 4,200,000 Indonesian Rupiah. Stack of bills three inches thick. Paid the total hotel bill and still have a million, two hundred thousand left. Hmmm. Goes fast, just like in Canada and I have the hotel all to myself, I'm the only one here. 29 rooms, 10 hotel employees and me.

In case you're not clear on what 3,000,000 Rupiah's paid for, here's the breakdown. 13 nights in a nice hotel and 4 car transfers, 2 of those were 4 hours each. Converted to U.S, that's $351.00. Nobody can complain about that.

Hours later after driving on what I consider one of the worst highway and secondary road systems I've ever been on, I got my first glimpse of Krakatoa offshore shrouded in rain and fog. It doesn't look so scary.

Got to the hotel at 4:00 pm and now if my calculations are correct, total traveling time is around 37 hours and now I'm seriously feeling it. I lay there the longest time not really sure what day or time it was. Jet lag finally caught up me. I got up at 7:00 am on March 10th. How much sleep? No clue.

March 10th

"...if tourists start getting knocked off..."

So now I'm awake and coherent (I think) and want some concrete details of my possible camping experience. And concrete details I got. One can only learn so much from the internet and emailing back and forth, I find sitting in front of the actual person is best and Deni the hotel manager is it.

The deal is because it's the rainy season, access to the volcano is somewhat limited unless you don't mind getting wet (I don't) and now I find out park police/rangers (Krakatau is designated as a park) seriously patrol the area and long term camping there will never happen unless you can slip by them and they don't spot you camped out. Get caught, penalties are severe, so I'm told. What that means, I don't know. If that means time in an Indonesian jail, well that would be bad.

I guess it's not healthy for Indonesian tourism if tourists start getting knocked off by a slightly overactive volcano. The only real deal presented to me that I see as workable is camping out two days/one night with proper permits, which means more cash for the government. What else is new!

The only bright side of this is Deni is going to try and arrange that we can camp out the one night right at the base of the actual volcano, not one of the off-islands. Now that would be awesome.

That's all I've got for today. Sleep time at 2:00 pm cause in my mind it's still really 2:00 am. By the time I get the jet lag sorted out, I'll be back in my own bed at home and have to go through this all over again.

March 11th

"…earthquake and tsunami…"

All set up now for going to the volcano next Tuesday at 10:00 am and we can camp out overnight at its base and also can climb to the top if it's not hardcore active. Talked to the boat guy who's in charge of all this and who's been there many times. He sees no problem in doing what I need to do, but camping there for an extended period would break me cash wise. This two day/1 night only camping experience costs 4 million RP. In U.S that's app $469.00. That's more than the 13 nights in the hotel.

Woke up at 5 am or so listening to the Muslim prayer chants or songs that are piped in somehow all through the town. It reminds me of being in Cairo, Egypt in 1990. I listened to that every morning. So that's why El Presidente relocated here.

I sat in the lobby having a tea when on the television came the news of an earthquake and tsunami that hit Japan. All countries in the area are on high alert, including this one. Ohoh!

March 12th

"...Indonesian people are not exactly huge..."

The alert for neighboring countries around Japan had been lifted, but the damage there is incredible. And I get to fly into Tokyo and spend 10 hours there in nine days.

I decided to take a bus up to a place called Labuan app 10 km from the hotel. There is supposedly a bazaar of some type, a bank and a supermarket. To grab one of these "buses" all you have to do is stand on the side of the road and wave one down, which I did.

I climbed into what appears to be a Toyota type minivan that's been slightly converted. By that I mean the sliding side passenger door has been replaced by a half normal type door which is always left open and in the back, it's been gutted and two small bench seats have been installed that run from the driver's seat to the back of the van and from the open door to the back of the van as well.

Off we go, I'm the only one in it so far. The driver stopped occasionally to pick up and drop people off. They paid nothing or next to nothing from what I can see. Tourists are expected to pay full price, which depending on who you talk to varies wildly. I picked a price of 5000 RP which in U.S $ is app .57 cents. Not bad for a 10 km ride. And you pay when you get to where you're going, not when they pick you up.

So I actually got dropped off where I wanted to go. If you read my Costa Rica taxi and bus stories you know that's rare, for me anyway. So I'm six feet tall and at this point in time, 255 lbs and getting in and out of this thing is not easy. I climbed out backwards and into total chaos. I have never seen anything like this in my life. Shanty shack stores one after another and I'm deluged by people

171

wanting to sell me stuff and offer me a ride somewhere, either on a pedal type rickshaw, scooter or motorcycle.

"No thank you," I said more times than I can count. It's unbelievable. I managed to make my way to the bank which was closed because new paver stones were being installed at the entrance. "Come back Monday" I'm told. I think that's what he said.

So that's a bust. Next stop is the supermarket. I only came here to buy some fruit, cheese, buns maybe and flip-flops. This supermarket has none of what I'm looking for except the flip-flops. I bought the biggest ones which barely fit because don't forget, Indonesian people are not exactly huge. They are for the most part, tiny and all the shoes and clothing items for sale reflect that.

"...two guys hanging out the open door..."

Time to get out of here I'm thinking so I left the market and I swear to God, could not walk more than six feet at a time without being stopped by someone wanting to sell me something. I have a fair amount of patience, but was losing if fast. Spotted another of these "buses," jumped in and all I'm thinking is "get me out of here."

Off we go, I'm the only passenger so far and then we start picking people up. First pickup is eight schoolgirls all dressed in the usual Muslim clothing. Only skin visible is the face and hands. As they climb on I'm moving farther to the back.

So now you have to use your imagination here. By the time I was dropped off at the hotel in this Toyota type minivan same as described earlier, there was two people in the single person passenger seat, one sitting on top of the other. There were two guys hanging out the open door, eight Muslim schoolgirls on the benches and me jammed in the back corner. I wonder how many religious rules were broken there. And on top of all that, I'm the first one that has to get off.

That was an experience all on its own and I get to do it again on Monday, because I still have to go the bank. Into the hotel I went and straight to bed which lasted about 10 minutes. It's two in the afternoon and I had asked yesterday if I could get my clothes washed. "No problem," I'm told. Knock/knock/knock at my door, I opened it and the cook is standing there who is also the laundry woman I guess.

I made the mistake of giving her everything except the pants I had on. Everything! I figured I'd have them back in a couple of hours. Wrong! The rest of the day I'm walking around in my new flip-flops, my only pair of pants and my winter jacket from Canada. Did I look the fool or what!

I gave her my clothes at around two in the afternoon and as I'm writing this at 6:00 am the next day, I still don't have them back. Nobody told me they didn't have a dryer. Duhh!!

March 13th

Finally got my clothes back at noon and I retired the winter jacket quick! It's Sunday and there are lots of people around. It's a slow day here and nothing is really happening. Just counting down to volcano departure day.

March 14th

"...I was on the wrong one..."

Back to Labuan today. I have to hit the bank and convert my money for the volcano trip tomorrow. I found out that bank I went to Friday does not change money. WHAT!!

I was directed to a little dingy place that does. I'm gonna get robbed for sure. Anyway, I went to this hole in the wall place and was pleasantly surprised that it was a legit establishment. I converted my money, shook hands with the two owners and left.

I jumped on the first "bus" I came across and off we go. I had just committed the number one cardinal sin. I didn't ask where the "bus" was going. Five minutes into the trip I knew I was on the wrong one. GOD!!

Once I'd made it clear to the driver I'd taken the wrong bus, he informed the others on the bus of my stupidity and they laughed and laughed. Well, I got a one hour tour of I have no idea where, but the scenery was lovely. I'm back in Labuan again so let's try this again.

Success! I'm back at my hotel feeling very tired and dumb. Paid Deni for the volcano trip and that's that. All these years of thinking about this and tomorrow it becomes a reality. Oh Boy.

Day 1

"...Sharks, sharks everywhere..."

Left Carita beach at 9:30 am and it took approximately two hours to get to the Krakatoa islands. It was raining hard and the sea was rough. Feels kinda strange going on this trip with three other people knowing I have to camp out overnight with them. I'm so used to doing this on my own. Sort of.

We stopped after entering a fog bank, couldn't see anything around us. The boat driver was going strictly by compass. We waited a long time until the fog began to clear and suddenly there it was, Krakatoa. They asked me what I wanted to do and I asked if we could circle Anak Krakatau, which is the volcano that popped out of the ocean in the 1920's.

So we circled the island and I had the camera and camcorder going steady. I'd come a long way for this and wanted to photograph everything. Looking at the volcano, I started to wonder if I could actually climb this thing. It sure looked big and it was smoldering everywhere. I'll decide tomorrow.

The island across the way was the one I had originally picked to camp out on if I had managed to be able to camp here alone. Satellite photos are of course shot from above and looking it from the water level, the spots I had picked were impossible to get to. They were just straight drop-offs to the water. So that plan would never have worked.

The boat driver started heading for the beach to what I now see are prearranged camping areas. Looks like there are two of them. He picked one and we anchored the boat and went ashore. The beaches are all jet black from pulverized lava. Feels like regular sand under the feet, but start wading into the water and the lava is not so broken up. 15 feet from the shoreline and your walking on mini boulders and then the bottom just drops off. I took one step too many and glug, glug, disappeared.

That's enough of that, I'm thinking and back to solid ground I go. Sharks. sharks everywhere I'm sure. The boys say no, but I don't believe them. For once I took my brothers advice.

I sat on the shore taking in the scenery while the boys set up camp. Hmmm. There may be some advantages to this after all. After a while I thought I'd go and take a look at this campsite of ours. Not bad actually. Two tents under a canopy, which was a terrific idea, cause it's still raining. Hard!

One of the boys started chopping up wood for a fire. How's he going to get and keep that burning in this rain is all I'm thinking. No sooner did that thought cross my mind, the rain stopped.

One of the other guys is the head chef and he was running around setting up a mini kitchen next to the tents. I turned around and a fire is going. Wow! These guys are good. By this time it was around five in the afternoon and after making us all some tea, the chef started preparing dinner.

I went into my tent to transfer the pictures I'd taken so far to my netbook, just to make sure they looked ok. I can't afford no mistakes, there's only one shot at this. No sooner had I hooked everything up, the boat driver starting yelling from the shore. I looked out the tent flap and he's motioning us to come over. "Bring your camera," he's yelling at me I think. I did, ran down to the shore and he's pointing up. Overhead is a giant brown cloud of smoke the volcano had just belched out. It was drifting right over our heads. The smell of sulphur was everywhere. How great is this. Deni took a picture of me with the cloud behind me.

I sat on the beach watching the cloud of smoke drift away; the sun was just starting to go down so I wandered back to the campsite. The next thing I know, dinner is served. Fish grilled on the open fire. rice, vegetables and fruit for dessert. It was a very nice way to end the day, and it took me back to the big shots I met in Antigua. They had the same deal going with their quarter million plus rented yachts.

We all sat around the campfire in darkness talking as best we could with Deni the hotel manager doing the translations. The day finally caught up with me and I said goodnight to the boys and went to bed.

I laid in there listening to the deafening sounds of the insects all night. Slept a little I think, not real sure. When you're on a volcanic island for only one night, who wants to sleep. But twice as I was lying there, the insect noises would stop suddenly and I could feel the ground rumbling under me. Wasn't earthquake movement, but I could definitely feel it. Cool!

Day 2

"...six to eight foot long lizard..."

Woke up early, still thinking how disconcerting it is to be half asleep last night and feel the entire island rumbling under me as I'm lying on my back. Quite disconcerting indeed.

Climbed out of the tent to find the fire had actually stayed lit all night. Guess one of the boys looked after it. I heard them now and then moving about. Also heard lots of other things moving about.

The fella that doubles as the cook got breakfast going. Having a cup of tea made for me at 6 am was certainly a new experience. Breakfast was an omelet and rice. I'd decided due to my knees not being what they used to be and the constant steam coming from various spots near the craters edge, not to climb up this thing. Views from a distance are going to have to be good enough.

The boys started packing up and I went for a very shallow swim. Enough with the shallow swimming, that's no fun whatsoever. I walked back to the half packed up campsite, when somebody shouted and was pointing to the bushes next to us. The rest of us turned to look and about 10 feet away was a six to eight foot long lizard. It was either a Komodo dragon or a monitor lizard so I'm told.

Everybody started backing up at the sight of that thing, I grabbed my camcorder, and as I started it up, the lizard came right into the campsite, with its very long tongue or whatever you call it darting in and out. It came to within three feet of us as we all stood dead still. Somebody moved slightly and the thing just darted away, looking back at us all the while. Such exciting stuff but where did it come from?

"...how prehistoric it looked..."

The boys continued packing and I grabbed all my stuff, put it in the boat and swam out in the water one final time. As I was standing out there with the water up to my neck, two of the lizards (how many are there here?) came onto the beach and walked right into the surf. They swim? Guess that's how they got here in the first place. As they waded in, I waded out. Screw this!

All packed and off we go. We circled the island again and then we went over to the location of the old volcano, the remnants of the one that erupted and exploded out of the ocean 128 years ago. As we approached, I was kind of taken aback at how prehistoric it looked and the bird noises were deafening. We went ashore and other than a small narrow strip of beach, behind me it was almost straight up. The peak of the island was shrouded in clouds.

Had a quick lunch, more shallow swimming and then we packed up and headed back to Carita Beach. The water was rougher on the way back and the sun had been out for quite a while. I started feeling the burning on my head and all other exposed skin. I ended up with a wicked sunburn.

I sat in the boat and watched as Anak Krakatau faded into the distance, thinking of the history here and what future history will be witnessed and written someday. If that thing goes up like the original Krakatau did in 1883, the effects here will be catastrophic. Over 35,000 people killed back then, I wonder what the populations of the coastal areas are now.

March 17th

Oh, I'm so sunburned! Only thing I did today was grab one of those mini buses to Labuan to change some more money. By my calculations, I need to change $27 US into local currency and that should be enough to see me through. So I did that, jumped on the first bus I found and back to Carita Beach I go. Not much else.

March 18th

Didn't do a damn thing!

March 19th

I'm leaving for Jakarta tomorrow morning, so I started packing early. Checked out the status of Narita airport in Tokyo, and according to the news, it's a mad house there. The tsunami was bad enough, now there's a problem with one of their nuclear power plant reactors leaking. So many are trying to get out of Japan, the airport is inundated with people. And I get to fly into that giant mess on Mar 21st. Great!

I contacted my travel agent and he told me to scrap my plan of leaving the airport and taking a train into Tokyo for a few hours. I have a 10 ½ hour layover there. Anything serious happens while I'm away from the airport, I'll be stuck there for God knows how long.

Anyway I'll worry about that when the time comes. Tonight is my last night here and I'll enjoy it as best I can.

March 20th

"…a 600 ton block of coral…"

My driver for Jakarta, El Presidente, is here. I said goodbye to all my new friends at the Sunset View Hotel in Carita and off we went. My only request on the drive back was to stop at a place called Anyer. The effects of the volcanic eruption are still visible there. By that, I mean there was a lighthouse there called the Fourth Point Lighthouse and during the Krakatoa event, it was completely destroyed.

The story goes: "And as the 120 foot tidal wave or tsunami, as they are now called, came ashore, it brought with it a 600 ton block of coral. As fate would have it, the coral and the lighthouse became one, so to speak. And the lighthouse was no more. All that's left from that time is the original pad the lighthouse was built on."

Visiting this spot was obviously on my "to do list." An hour after we left the hotel, the lighthouse that was rebuilt in 1885 came into view and we stopped. I walked over and stood on the pad of the original lighthouse and directly behind me was the new lighthouse. But the thing I tried to imagine the most standing there was what it must have felt like for the lighthouse keeper and his family to have stood there and watched all these events happening. The lighthouse keeper survived, his wife and child did not.

Standing on that pad, out in the Sundra Strait I could see the old and new Krakatau clear as a bell. It doesn't look that far from this vantage point. And again, as I did a few days ago, all I could think of was what will happen to all the people here if Krakatau goes up again.

We jumped back in the car and before I know it, we're back in Jakarta and I'm back in the same hotel I started this journey from. My head for some reason is just throbbing now and its time, I think, for some sleep and silence.

Into bed at three in the afternoon with a raging headache and just down the hall from me? Some type of live band with a wedding or get together of some kind going on. Pillows over my head as well as under and the next thing I know it's............

March 21st

"...Happy birthday dad..."

It's my last day here. Off to the airport at seven pm tonight to catch my flight to Tokyo. What kind of madhouse will I find there? No clue.

Today for me anyway, is a happy and a sad day. Today is my tenth anniversary of sobriety. Who would have thought I would make it his long. Nobody around me I'm sure. But I knew I would, enough was enough!

Also, today would have been my father's 90th birthday. He missed it by four months. Happy birthday dad, and as I said in the dedication, you are missed by many.

I spent the time up to seven pm writing, sleeping and searching for a store that sells peanuts. President Mubarak showed up as scheduled and off to the airport I go. I was also successful in the peanut search. My next stop is Tokyo. With everything that's happened there since March 11th, it should be interesting.

Plane left as scheduled at 10:05 pm. It was a Boeing 777 which seats maybe 300+? I counted 40 people on it. Guess everybody's leaving Japan and nobody wants to go there. That's certainly understandable. Every person on the plane had a row of seats to themselves, which was great. I just stretched out across three seats and fell asleep.

March 22nd

"…that's truly it…"

Arrived at seven am and after a confusing time finding out where I had to go, I finally found the Air Canada check-in counter. It opens at 2:10 pm and right now it's eight am. Gonna be a long day. And it was! Two mini earthquakes later and I'm off on my final leg of this journey back to Canada. Well, not so fast. Seems the Air Canada flight crews aren't staying in Tokyo anymore due to the leaky reactor 200 km up north from here. Radiation from that plant is drifting this way and everybody's scared.

So I have one more stop on my way. Osaka, and when we landed, nobody was allowed off the plane. That's two cities in Japan I never got to visit.

The flight crews swapped out and we are finally on our way. From the time I walked out the front door of the hotel in Jakarta, to walking into the front door of where I live, 33 hours had passed and 12 time zones and the

International date line crossed again. 66 hours in total spent in airports and airplanes. Very grueling indeed and I guess this time "that's truly it."

Aftermath

I didn't do this trip to lose any weight. I knew camping out for an extended period of time on the volcano most likely would not be an option and I was right. Camping out one night and two days on it with a cook in attendance isn't going to help.

I was pleasantly surprised though when I got home and I weighed exactly what I did when I left, 255lbs. Maybe that's the weight I'm going to have to accept as my goal weight. I don't want it to be, but its sure better than 315 and the best thing is it only took eight years. Never said I was a quick study.

In my head I want to step on the scale one day and see it read 199. Will it ever happen? My feeling now is the answer is no. But, never say never. My first step though is to try and stay around the 250 mark. I'm sure that will be a struggle in itself. And when the stop smoking day rolls around, which I know it will, then there's going to be trouble. This trip only gets a ¼ point, cause while I didn't lose anything, I didn't put any weight back on either.

Final Score: 3 ¾ out of 8 attempts.
(Almost a 50 % success rate.)

Google "Krakatoa: The Last Days." It's a docudrama that I've watched several times and there are links to clips on YouTube that you might find interesting.

Aftermath Part 2

Well, the quit smoking day finally arrived, June 25th 2011. I had kept my weight in the 250-260 range since I'd come back from Krakatoa three months ago.

And horror of horrors, what was the result? Exactly what I knew it would be. The weight just piled back on. And on. And on. I ended up back to where I was in the July 2003. Talk about going full circle!

As I write this now on September 16th 2012. I haven't smoked in 15 months. Do I feel any better? Absolutely NOT!! My doctor has told me better to be a little heavier and not smoke. A little heavier???

I figure I'll get a 12 month grace period before the "you gotta lose that weight" lecture starts. I was right, 12 months later and everybody is singing the same song. Diet time, diet time. What a crock.

That's it, thanks for plowing thru this and I'll try and keep you updated with weights and pictures through the sites below.

Score: Reset to 0. DAMN!!!!!

facebook.com/shannon.dietfailures
Website: www.dietfailures.com
Twitter: @dietfailures